COLOR GUIDE

Gynecology

Janice Rymer MD MRCOG FRNZCOG
Senior Lecturer/Consultant in Obstetrics and Gynaecology
UMDS, Guy's and St Thomas' Hospital
London

Andrew N. J. Fish MD MRCOG
Consultant in Obstetrics and Gynaecology
Brighton Health Care
Brighton

Michael Chapman MD FRCOG
Professor of Obstetrics and
Gynaecology
St George's Hospital
Kogarah
Sydney

SECOND EDITION

U.S. Advisor

Martin P. R. Walker MD
Assistant Professor of Reproductive Medicine
UCSD Medical Center
University of California, San Diego, CA

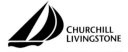

CHURCHILL
LIVINGSTONE

EDINBURGH LONDON NEW YORK PHILADELPHIA SAN FRANCISCO
SYDNEY TOKYO 1997

CHURCHILL LIVINGSTONE

© Harcourt Brace and Company Limited

⚓ is a registered trademark of Harcourt Brace and Company Limited

J. Rymer, A. N. J. Fish and M. Chapman have asserted their right under the Copyright, Designs and Patents Act, 1988, to be identified as Authors of this work.

Adapted from Colour Guide Gynaecology Second Edition by J. Rymer, A. Fish and M. Chapman

ISBN 0 443 05878 4

Library of Congress Cataloging in Publication Data
A catalog record for this book is available from the Library of Congress.

Medical knowledge is constantly changing. As new information becomes available, changes in treatment, procedures, equipment, and the use of drugs become necessary. The authors and the publishers have, as far as it is possible, taken care to ensure that the information given in this text is accurate and up to date. However, readers are strongly advised to confirm that the information, especially with regard to drug usage, complies with current legislation and standards of practice.

Produced by Addison Wesley Longman China Limited, Hong Kong.
SWTC/01

The publisher's policy is to use **paper manufactured from sustainable forests**

For Churchill Livingstone

Publisher: Tim Horne
Project editor: James Dale
U.S. copy-editor: Donna Regen
Project controller: Kay Hunston
Design direction: Erik Bigland

Acknowledgments

We are grateful to the following for providing some of the illustrations for this book: Sir John Dewhurst, Dr. R. J. S. Harris, Dr. E. Lombardi, Dr. J. Robinson, Mr. D. H. Oram, Dr. S. Thorpe, Dr. P. Greenhouse, Miss M. Hooper, Dr. S. Barton, Dr. R. Jelley, Mr. R. Forman, Dr. I. Fogelman, Dr. C. Brown, Mr. E. Versi, Dr. F. Mitchell, Mr. A. Cutner, The Royal College of Surgeons, and Gower Medical Publishing. We would especially like to thank Dr. Jo Rosenthal for reading the scripts and providing useful criticisms. We are indebted to the photographic departments of Guy's Hospital, Royal London Hospital, and Brighton Health Care.

Contents

1 / Making a gynecologic diagnosis

History

A thorough history is essential to make an accurate gynecologic diagnosis.

Setting

The setting for the interview should ensure privacy and comfort for the woman, who should not be asked to undress before being interviewed.

Content

Specific information should be gathered regarding:
- parity
- last menstrual period
- length of the menstrual cycle
- contraceptive use
- date of the last cervical smear

The presenting complaint should be clearly defined and put in the context of the previous obstetric and gynecologic history (Fig. 1). It is important to record information about sexual activity: duration of the present sexual relationship and any recent change in sexual partner. In cases of suspected infection, it is mandatory to ask about the symptoms of the partner(s).

Examination: Positions

Positions

A pelvic examination can be performed with the patient either in the dorsal position or in the left lateral position (Figs. 2 and 3). Sims position, which is similar to the coma position, may also be used. In the dorsal position, the external genitalia are easily inspected, with particular reference to the vulva, labia, clitoris, and urethra.

HEALTH AUTHORITY	Surname	Mr Mrs Miss	Unit No.								
			D.O.B.				
HOSPITAL CONSULTANT	First Names		

Date	Notes
	Age Parity Last Menstrual Period –/–/–
	Cycle / Contraception Last Cervical Smear –/–/–
	Presenting Problem
	Previous Obstetric and Gynaecological History
	Previous Medical History
	Social History / Family History Drugs
	Allergies
	Clinical Findings

G Y N A E C O L O G Y

Fig. 1 History sheet.

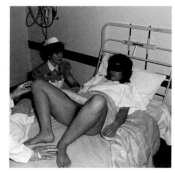

Fig. 2 Examination in the dorsal position.

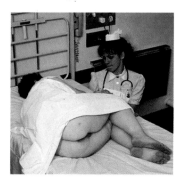

Fig. 3 Patient in the left lateral position.

Examination: Instruments and techniques

Bivalve speculum

A bivalve speculum is used to inspect the cervix and the vaginal walls (Fig. 4). It is also used when taking cervical smears and endocervical swabs.

Bimanual examination

A bimanual examination is performed to assess the pelvic organs. One or two fingers of the right hand are inserted into the vagina and used to elevate and steady the uterus and adnexa so that the left hand on the abdomen can feel the pelvic organs (Fig. 5). The size, position (anteverted, axial, or retroverted), and mobility of the uterus are determined, together with the presence of tenderness and/or masses in the fornices. *Cervical excitation* is defined as tenderness that arises in one or other adnexum when the broad ligament is stretched by movement of the cervix with the examining fingers.

Sims speculum

The left lateral position facilitates the use of a Sims speculum (Fig. 6). This instrument was originally designed for displaying vesicovaginal fistulas. It is now more often used in the assessment of uterovaginal prolapse. One end of the speculum is inserted into the vagina, and gentle traction is applied backward. The anterior vaginal wall is thus visualized. To view the posterior vaginal wall, a pair of sponge-holding forceps is inserted to retract the anterior vaginal wall while the Sims speculum is slowly withdrawn.

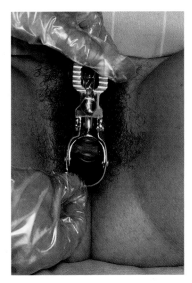

Fig. 4 Examination with a bivalve speculum.

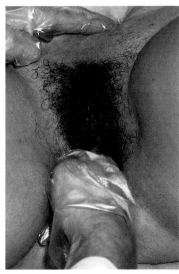

Fig. 5 Bimanual examination.

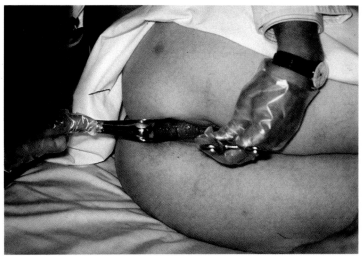

Fig. 6 Examination using Sims speculum.

Taking a cervical smear

The cervix should be clearly visualized by using a bivalve speculum. The narrow point of the wooden spatula is inserted into the endocervical canal so that the lip rests against the cervix (Fig. 7). It is then rotated through 360 degrees, keeping in firm contact with the cervix, and then removed. The material collected on the spatula is spread evenly on a microscope slide (Fig. 8), which is immediately immersed in fixative (3% acetic acid in 95% alcohol). The American College of Obstetrics and Gynecology recommends that endocervical cells be obtained by using a cytobrush or cotton swab before ectocervical scraping using an Ayre's spatula.

Indications

All sexually active women should have smears taken at 3-year intervals.

Taking microbiologic swabs

High vaginal swabs are taken from the posterior fornix by using a bivalve speculum. The cotton-tipped swab is placed in the appropriate transport medium.

Indications

High vaginal swabs are used to detect lower genital tract pathogens (e.g., *Candida albicans* or *Trichomonas vaginalis*) that give rise to symptoms such as discharge and vulval irritation. Endocervical swabs are used to detect pathogens that may spread to the upper genital tract and cause pelvic inflammatory disease (e.g., *Chlamydia trachomatis* and *Neisseria gonorrhoeae*). These bacteria infect columnar epithelium. The microbiologic swab should be inserted into the endocervical canal (Fig. 9), agitated, and withdrawn. It should then be placed in the appropriate transport medium.

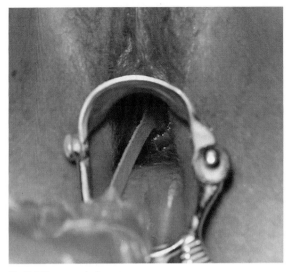

Fig. 7 Taking a cervical smear.

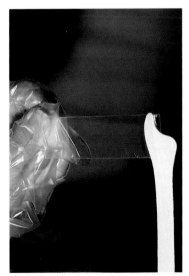

Fig. 8 Spreading the smear on a microscope slide.

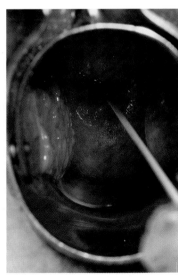

Fig. 9 Taking an endocervical swab.

Colposcopy

Indications

All women who have had cervical smears showing mild dyskaryosis that does not resolve spontaneously, or those women with a single smear showing moderately or severely dyskaryotic cells, should undergo colposcopy.

Description

The colposcope (Fig. 10) is a binocular microscope. An illuminated, three-dimensional view of the cervix is obtained, magnified between 6 and 40 times (Fig. 11). This technique identifies both the severity of the abnormality giving rise to an abnormal smear and also its position on the cervix. Hence, it allows the clinician to assess the suitability for local ablative therapy.

Technique

The patient is examined in the lithotomy position, and a bivalve speculum is used to expose the cervix. A further cervical smear is usually taken prior to the colposcopic examination. Cotton wool swabs are then used to clean mucus off the cervix before applying 5% acetic acid to stain the abnormal areas white (acetowhite). If the upper limit of the transformation zone lies within the endocervical canal, forceps may be useful in exposing the whole area (Fig. 12). If the upper limit of the transformation zone cannot be visualized, then the examination must be considered incomplete. This occurs in <10% of women aged 25 years or younger, but in >30% of women older than the age of 40 years.

Punch biopsy forceps can be used to obtain a sample from colposcopically abnormal areas to make a histologic diagnosis. Once the results of this are known, ablative treatment such as SEMM cautery or laser can be applied. Loop excision of the transformation zone is being increasingly used. For women with moderate or severely dyskaryotic smears and colposcopic changes consistent with this, the treatment process removes the abnormality and produces a good sample for histologic analysis, enabling assessment and treatment at one visit (see and treat).

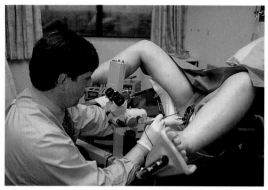

Fig. 10 Colposcopy clinic.

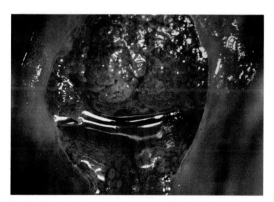

Fig. 11 Colpophotograph of a normal cervix.

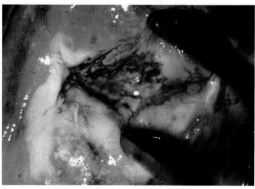

Fig. 12 Exposing the squamocolumnar junction.

Ultrasound

Description

Ultrasonography records high-frequency sound waves as they are reflected from anatomic structures. Ultrasound waves are mechanical waves beyond the scope of hearing. When they are directed toward media of differing densities, the sound waves spread out with differing velocities. Echoes arise at the interfaces between these media, and the greater the density differences, the greater the intensity of the echoes. This echo signal is measured and converted into a clinical picture of the area under examination. Thus, for good visualization, there must be an air-free coupling of the transducer to the abdomen. Ultrasound is a simple and painless procedure that has no known ill effects. The ultrasonographer and patient can look at the ultrasound image together (Fig. 13).

Various probes are now available (Fig. 14). If an abdominal probe is used, the scan is performed with a full bladder, which provides a sonographic "window." A vaginal probe eliminates the need to have a full bladder, which is especially useful in early pregnancy.

Indications

Ultrasonography is useful in almost any pelvic abnormality as all structures can usually be demonstrated, except in very obese women. Blood flow to various organs can be demonstrated by using color Doppler techniques (Fig. 15).

The first sign of an intrauterine pregnancy can be detected in the 5th week as a small, sharply outlined cavity, which is the gestational sac. Between the 7th and 8th weeks, embryonic structures can be visualized as distinct echoes, and the fetal heart can be seen beating.

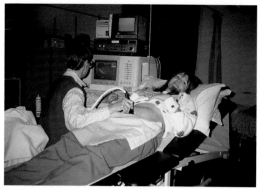

Fig. 13 Abdominal ultrasound being performed.

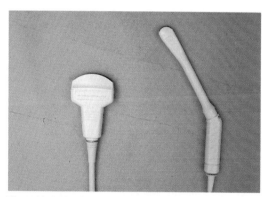

Fig. 14 Vaginal and abdominal ultrasound probes.

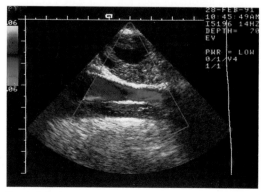

Fig. 15 Color Doppler ultrasound illustrating normal ovarian blood flow.

Hysterosalpingography

Description

Hysterosalpingography (HSG) is a radiographic method of assessing fallopian tube patency and demonstrating structural abnormalities of the uterine cavity.

Indications

HSG will show whether the fallopian tubes are patent. If not, the area in which the tubes are blocked can be identified. It will not give information concerning the condition of the pelvis (i.e., the presence of peritubular adhesions and/or pelvic distortion, which may impair fertility even though the tubes are patent).

Technique

HSG is usually performed without anesthetic in the radiology department. A bivalve speculum is used to expose the cervix, which is cannulated to enable radiopaque dye to be injected into the uterine cavity. The procedure is viewed by using an image intensifier and recorded on film (Fig. 16).

Hysteroscopy

Description and technique

Hysteroscopy is a method that enables visual examination of the uterine cavity. A hysteroscope is a telescope surrounded by a sheath. It is inserted into the uterine cavity through the cervix with the patient in the lithotomy position and under either local or general anesthesia.

Indications

Endometrial polyps, fibroids, and adhesions within the uterine cavity can be visualized hysteroscopically, together with different types of endometrium (e.g., normal, hyperplastic, atrophic, and malignant) (Figs. 17–19). It is also possible to use the hysteroscope to take endometrial biopsies, divide adhesions, and remove polyps and misplaced intrauterine contraceptive devices (IUCD). The endometrial lining can be removed by using an electrical resection loop or laser in women with menorrhagia. Submucous fibroids can also be removed in this way.

Complications

Complications of the procedure include perforation of the uterus, infection, and fluid overload (e.g., if fluid distension medium is used for endometrial resection).

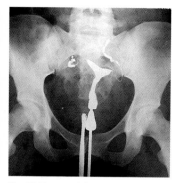

Fig. 16 Hysterosalpingogram outlining the uterine and tubal anatomy.

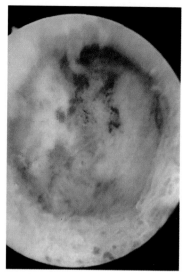

Fig. 17 Normal endometrium.

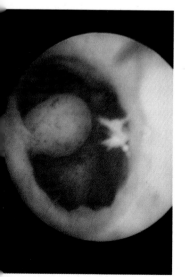

Fig. 18 Endometrial polyp.

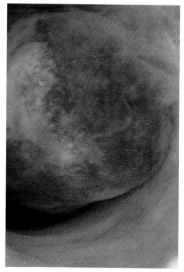

Fig. 19 Endometrial pedunculated fibroid.

Laparoscopy

Description

The laparoscope is essentially a telescope that is inserted into the abdominal cavity after it has been inflated with carbon dioxide. The direct view obtained allows the diagnosis of gynecologic disorders and surgery (Figs. 20 and 21) without laparotomy.

Technique

The procedure is almost invariably performed under general anesthesia with the patient paralyzed and ventilated. The patient is placed in position with the head down. The bladder is catheterized. A small incision is made at the umbilicus, and a Verres needle is inserted into the peritoneal cavity. Approximately 3 L of carbon dioxide are insufflated into the peritoneal cavity. The needle is withdrawn, and the laparoscopic trocar and cannula are inserted. The trocar is withdrawn and replaced with the laparoscope, which allows direct visualization of the pelvic organs (Fig. 22). If needed, further cannulas are inserted under direct laparoscopic vision, suprapubically or in either iliac fossa, to permit manipulation of pelvic organs and instrumentation for various surgical techniques.

Indications

These include pelvic pain, exclusion and treatment of ectopic pregnancy, infertility, sterilization, trauma, lost IUCD, and assisted conception techniques, as well as staging procedures for gynecologic cancer, including pelvic lymph node sampling. Operative laparoscopy now has many applications (e.g., the treatment of endometriosis either by laser ablation or diathermy excision, removal of benign ovarian cysts, removal of ovaries at vaginal hysterectomy). More advanced procedures include laparoscopically assisted vaginal hysterectomy, laparoscopic colposuspensions, and laparoscopic sacrocolpopexies.

Complications

Complications of the procedure include:
- pain, especially shoulder tip pain from CO_2 diaphragmatic irritation
- bleeding
- puncture of bladder, bowel
- misplacement of gas

There is a mortality rate of approximately 1 in 15,000.

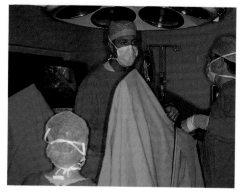

Fig. 20 In the operating room.

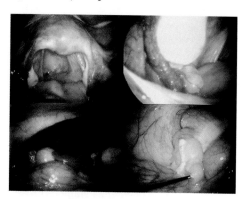

Fig. 21 Laparoscopic views of internal organs.

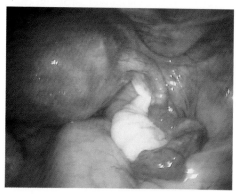

Fig. 22 Normal fallopian tube and ovary as seen with laparoscopy.

Congenital

Hydrocolpos

In this disorder, an imperforate membrane is situated immediately above the hymen. Above this obstruction, the vagina can become distended by fluid (Fig. 23). Hydrocolpos can present in the neonate as retention of urine, abdominal pain, and a lower abdominal swelling if there is a large quantity of fluid. The treatment is simple incision of the membrane to release the fluid.

Hematocolpos

The same situation as in hydrocolpos occurs in hematocolpos, except that the problem does not arise until puberty. The menstrual fluid is unable to be released and collects above the imperforate hymen, grossly expanding the vagina and even the uterus. The presenting symptoms may include abdominal pain, urinary retention, or a large abdominal mass. Vulval inspection will reveal a bulging bluish membrane that requires incision.

Fused labia

The labia minora become adherent to each other (Fig. 24), and it may appear as though the vagina is absent. The etiology is not known, but the condition is probably due to low estrogen levels. Application of estrogen cream usually results in spontaneous separation after 10–14 days.

Congenital abnormalities

The Müllerian (paramesonephric) ducts are the embryologic precursors of the fallopian tubes, uterus, and upper two-thirds of the vagina. The lower one-third of the vagina develops from the urogenital sinus. Various defects can occur during embryologic development (Fig. 25). These include failure of:

- development (e.g., no paramesonephric duct)
- paramesonephric duct canalization
- fusion of paramesonephric ducts
- median septum loss (Fig. 26)
- fundal dome development
- fusion of paramesonephric ducts with urogenital sinus
- transverse septum loss between paramesonephric system and urogenital sinus

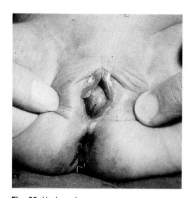

Fig. 23 Hydrocolpos.

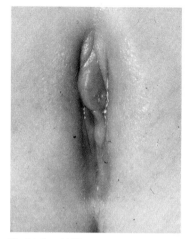

Fig. 24 Fused labia.

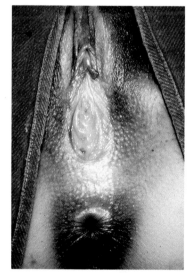

Fig. 25 Absent vagina—a congenital defect.

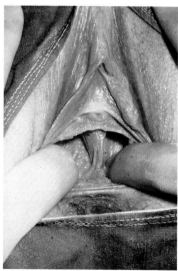

Fig. 26 Vaginal septum.

Problems in early childhood

Vulvovaginitis

This is the most common gynecologic problem in children. There are three factors that make the immature vagina susceptible to infection:

- lack of protective acid secretion
- contamination by stool and debris
- impaired mechanisms of immunity

The usual bacteriologic finding is of mixed bacterial flora. The child will complain of vulval soreness, discharge, or pain on micturition. Threadworm infestation can sometimes cause this condition.

Foreign bodies

These usually produce a purulent discharge or bleeding.

Botryoid sarcoma

Tumors are rare in childhood, but embryonal rhabdomyosarcoma is the most serious. It is often grapelike in appearance (Fig. 27) but may appear simply as a polyp. The tumor spreads extensively in the subepithelial tissues of the vagina or ectocervix. Chemotherapy is generally given prior to extended hysterectomy or vaginectomy (Fig. 28).

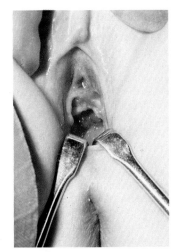

Fig. 27 Botryoid sarcoma at examination.

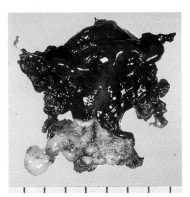

Fig. 28 Surgical specimen of botryoid sarcoma.

Sexual abuse

Children who have been sexually abused endure physical and psychological trauma. When sexual abuse is suspected, a thorough examination must be carried out by an experienced gynecologist. Swabs for sexually transmitted diseases must be taken from the vagina, cervix, and anus. Samples for semen should also be taken. Photographs should be taken if possible, and the signs of physical trauma accurately documented. The examinations are often performed under anesthesia.

Vulval bruising is common, and the hymen is often perforated (Fig. 29). Anal bruising must be looked for (Fig. 30), as well as anal dilation. The rest of the body must be searched for bruising or other signs of trauma. Fractures should be suspected. These children usually need admitting until the domestic situation has been thoroughly investigated. A multidisciplinary approach involving social workers, pediatricians, and gynecologists is usually adopted.

Female circumcision

This custom is still practiced, mainly in Africa. The extent of the procedure varies. If performed early in infancy, it is usually limited to trimming of the labia minora and the tip of the clitoris. Complications are rare. If the operation is carried out near puberty, hemorrhage and sepsis can be severe. Complete excision of the labia and minora is performed, and the denuded edges are encouraged to unite by strapping the thighs together, with a stick between the edges to allow passage of urine. The resulting scarring can be extreme and the urethra and vestibule hidden (Fig. 31). This deflects the urinary stream, causing chronic infection both of the surrounding skin and vagina. Intercourse may be impossible, and division of a skin bridge may be necessary. For vaginal delivery, an anterior episiotomy may be necessary. In obstructed labor, the fetus may be in the vagina for long enough to cause vaginal wall pressure necrosis.

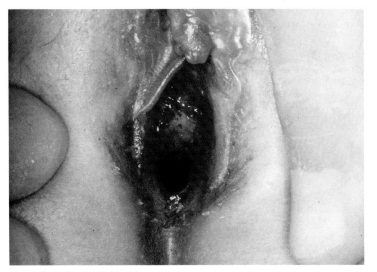

Fig. 29 Vaginal and vulval bruising.

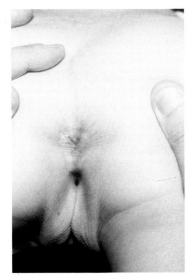

Fig. 30 Anal trauma.

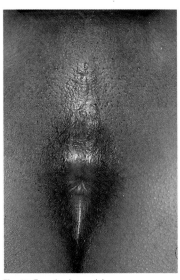

Fig. 31 Female circumcision.

Disorders of puberty

The hormonal changes of puberty are complex. Disordered function can reveal chromosomal, enzymatic, and structural abnormalities not obvious in childhood.

Turner syndrome

In Turner syndrome (Fig. 32), the absence of the one sex chromosome leads to ovarian dysgenesis, resulting in primary amenorrhea, short stature, and sexual infantilism. Alternatively, androgen-receptor defects with a normal XY complement lead to failure of masculinization and apparently normal, full breast development. Primary amenorrhea may be the first presentation of testicular feminization (Fig. 33).

5α reductase deficiency

In 5α reductase deficiency (Fig. 34), the lack of the enzyme likewise results in failure of masculinization of the external genitalia in the genotypic male child. However, at puberty the large increase in testosterone production by normal, internalized testes results in androgenization of the presumed female. The testes are removed, and estrogen replacement ensures a phenotypic female.

   Other problems include precocious puberty, as indicated by early thelarche or menarche, or delayed puberty in which hypothalamic maturation is pathologically late.

Intersex

Definition

An intersex is an individual in whom there is discordance between chromosomal, gonadal, internal genital, and phenotype sex, or the sex of rearing.

Clinical features

It may be declared at birth because of ambiguous external genitalia (Fig. 35), during childhood because of precocious puberty, or during adolescence because pubertal changes are inappropriate to presumed gender or because puberty fails to occur.

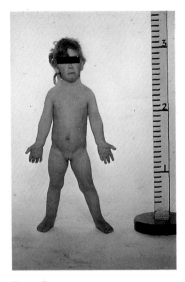

Fig. 32 Turner syndrome.

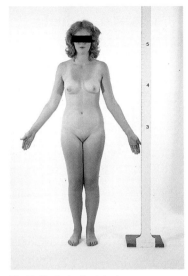

Fig. 33 Testicular feminization.

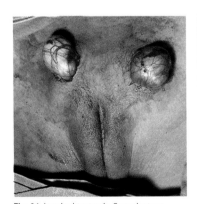

Fig. 34 Inguinal testes in 5α reductase deficiency.

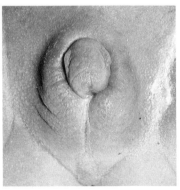

Fig. 35 Intersex.

4 / Menstrual cycle

Puberty

At puberty, the hypothalamus–pituitary–ovarian (PO) axis changes and gonadotropin-releasing hormone (GnRH) is secreted in a pulsatile fashion from the hypothalamus. This stimulates a pulsatile release of follicle-stimulating hormone (FSH) and luteinizing hormone (LH) from the anterior pituitary. Thereafter, FSH and LH are secreted in pulses every 70–220 min depending on the cycle phase. The release of the gonadotropins is regulated by the ovarian steroid feedback on the hypothalamus and pituitary.

Hormonal changes

At the beginning of each cycle (Fig. 36a), FSH stimulates growth in follicles, with one follicle becoming dominant. Estrogen production in the dominant follicle increases, leading to rising estradiol blood levels, which trigger the LH surge from the pituitary, in turn causing ovulation. This LH surge also stimulates the production of progesterone and prostaglandins in the follicle. The oocyte is then released from the follicle, which shrinks and becomes the progesterone-producing corpus luteum. Unless a pregnancy occurs, this regresses after about 10 days. If pregnancy occurs, the human chorionic gonadotropin (HCG) maintains the production of steroids from the corpus luteum until week 10 of pregnancy.

Endometrial changes

The endometrium in the first half of the cycle (Fig. 36b) responds to the estrogenic stimulation by growth of the glands and endometrial thickening. When progesterone is produced in the second half, the epithelium lining the glands develops vacuoles, and the glands and the spiral arterioles continue to grow. The stroma becomes edematous and under-goes decidualization. Falling levels of estrogen and progesterone cause constriction and dilation of the spiral arterioles; generalized vasoconstriction, ischemia, and cell disintegration occur, leading to release of lysosomal enzymes. Breakdown is halted by rising levels of estrogen from the next follicle. The cervix and vagina show changes in response to ovarian steroid output (Fig. 37).

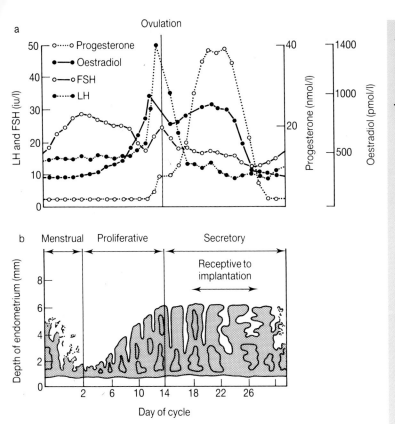

Fig. 36 Menstrual cycle. Hormonal changes (a). Endometrial changes (b).

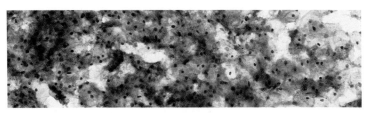

Fig. 37 Vaginal cytology showing estrogenic stimulation.

Amenorrhea

Amenorrhea is defined as the failure to menstruate. It can be classified as primary (menstruation fails to start) or secondary, which is defined as the cessation of periods for greater than 6 months. Amenorrhea may be due to the absence of the uterus as in an XY female, blockage of the outflow tract owing to an imperforate hymen, or endometrial disturbances (i.e., absence as in uterine scarring [Asherman syndrome], atrophy as in premature menopause, or hormonal imbalance as in polycystic ovarian syndrome).

Primary

Primary amenorrhea has been mentioned in disorders of puberty.

Secondary

The most common causes of secondary amenorrhea are hypothalamic suppression (Fig. 38), hyperprolactinemia (usually due to a prolactinoma, Fig. 39), or polycystic ovarian syndrome. Other causes include thyroid disease, adrenal disease, premature ovarian failure, and Sheehan syndrome. Sheehan syndrome is a form of hypopituitarism caused by postpartum ischemic necrosis of the anterior pituitary. The hypoplastic pituitary gland at pregnancy is more susceptible to hypotension, and severe postpartum hemorrhage may precipitate Sheehan syndrome.

Asherman syndrome should be suspected in women who have amenorrhea and have normal hormonal profiles with evidence of ovulation, particularly in women who have had some form of uterine surgery (e.g., termination of pregnancy or dilation and curettage [D&C]), which could precipitate the formation of intrauterine adhesions. Pregnancy and natural menopause are physiologic causes of amenorrhea. When a woman presents with secondary amenorrhea, pregnancy and natural menopause should always be considered.

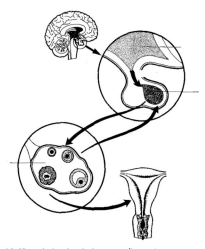

Fig. 38 Hypothalamic–pituitary–ovarian axis.

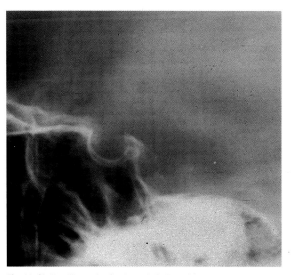

Fig. 39 Skull radiograph of enlarged pituitary fossa.

Dysfunctional uterine bleeding

Definition

Abnormal uterine bleeding after pelvic pathology has been excluded.

Etiology

Not known.

Classification

Cases can be divided into anovulatory or ovulatory.

Clinical features

The majority of patients will report heavy bleeding that may be regular or irregular. It is extremely difficult to make an accurate assessment of the amount of bleeding by relying on history alone. Quantitative measurement of blood loss can be made by collecting all the tampons and sanitary pads and using the alkalin hematin test.

On abdominal and pelvic examination, no abnormalities should be detected.

Investigations

To exclude pelvic pathology, a thorough pelvic assessment must be made, including cervical smear and endometrial biopsy (Fig. 40) if indicated. Ultrasound (Fig. 41), laparoscopy, hysteroscopy (Fig. 42), or color Doppler studies are investigations that may be used depending on the clinical situation.

Management

Anovulatory. In adolescents, the oral contraceptive pill will make the withdrawal bleeds lighter, regular, and less painful. In the perimenopausal woman, hormone replacement therapy or cyclical progestogens (after exclusion of uterine pathology) would be appropriate.

Ovulatory. Nonsteroidal anti-inflammatory drugs, the oral contraceptive pill, Danazol and antifibrinolytic drugs, or the progesterone-releasing intrauterine system (IUS) are the main options.

Hysterectomy or endometrial resection/ablation is used if the above measures fail.

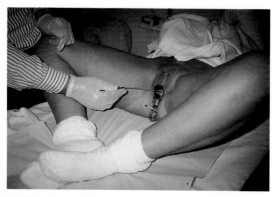

Fig. 40 Endometrial biopsy.

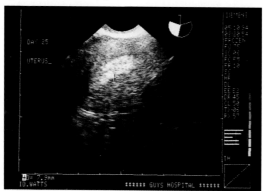

Fig. 41 Transvaginal ultrasound scan of endometrium.

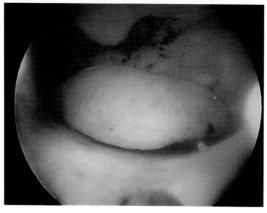

Fig. 42 Hysteroscopic view of an endometrial polyp.

5 / Contraception

"Natural" methods

Highest fertility occurs at ovulation: in a 28-day cycle, this occurs about 14 days after the last menstrual period. Sperm may survive in the genital tract for up to 7 days; therefore, to avoid conception, discontinue intercourse 1 week before ovulation is expected and recommence it not less than 2 days after ovulation has occurred. Ovulation may be predicted by:

- monitoring previous cycles (rhythm method)
- using the rise in body temperature with ovulation to determine the "safe period" (Fig. 43)
- assessing the cervical mucus, which becomes profuse and watery (spinbarkeit) at ovulation

The failure rates for these methods may be as high as 25 pregnancies per 100 women-years.

Coitus interruptus (removal of the penis from the vagina before ejaculation) is a widely used method of contraception; not particularly effective.

Barrier methods

Condoms. When used with a spermicide (e.g., Nonoxynol-9), condoms are an effective method of contraception, resulting in only 2–3 failures per 100 women-years. Condoms also act as a physical barrier to the transmission of many sexually transmitted infections; female condoms are also available (Fig. 44).

Caps. The diaphragm (Fig. 45) is the most commonly used; other types include cervical and vault caps. When used with spermicide, a diaphragm is as effective as a condom and spermicide. It consists of a thin latex rubber dome attached to a circular metal spring. The size required is determined during an examination by a physician. It should cover the cervix, with the anterior edge of the diaphragm lying behind the symphysis pubis and the posterior edge in the posterior fornix. It should be inserted prior to intercourse and should not be removed for at least 6 h afterward.

Others. Disposable sponges are not available in the United States. ➡

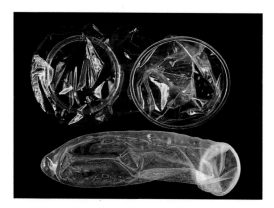

Fig. 43 Temperature chart—ovulatory biphasic pattern. Temperature rise follows ovulation and persists until just prior to menstruation.

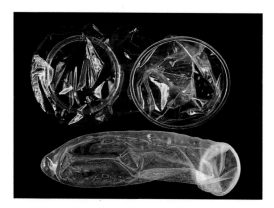

Fig. 44 Female condoms.

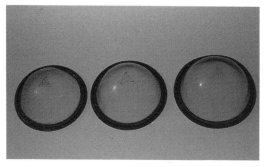

Fig. 45 Diaphragms.

Combined oral contraceptive pills. These contain both estrogen and progesterone (Fig. 46). They are taken cyclically for 21 days with a 7-day break. During the "pill-free week," a withdrawal bleed is experienced. The combined pill acts on the hypothalamus and pituitary, causing inhibition of GnRH, FSH, and LH by negative feedback, thus preventing ovulation. The endometrium is also rendered unsuitable for implantation. The progesterone element of the combined pill makes the cervical mucus impenetrable to sperm and may also interfere with fallopian tube function. The combined pill should not be used by women with hormone-dependent tumors (breast, endometrium, trophoblast). Thromboembolism, arterial disease, valvular heart disease, focal migraine, clotting abnormalities, and liver disease are all contraindications to pill usage. Smoking, hypertension, and diabetes are considered "relative contraindications". The combined pill is the most effective reversible method of contraception currently available.

Progesterone-only pills. These do not necessarily inhibit ovulation; they act on the endometrium, the endocervical mucus, and the fallopian tubes. Progesterone-only preparations should be taken at the same time every day, without any breaks. The maximal effect on cervical mucus is seen 4–6 h after taking the pills. Even with good compliance, progesterone-only pills are less effective than combined pills.

Depot progestogen injections. Used in sufficiently high doses, these will:
- inhibit ovulation
- render the endometrium atrophic
- thicken the cervical mucus

This form of contraception is effective, safe, convenient, and reversible. Some women will, however, suffer from weight gain and bleeding irregularities.

Norplant. Six rods inserted under the skin give contraception for up to 5 years (Fig. 47). Side effects include irregular and prolonged bleeding and amenorrhea. ➡

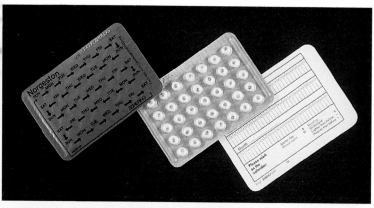

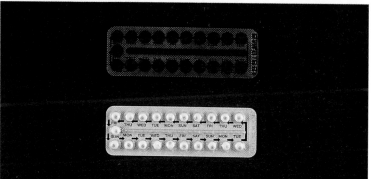

Fig. 46 Oral contraceptive pills.

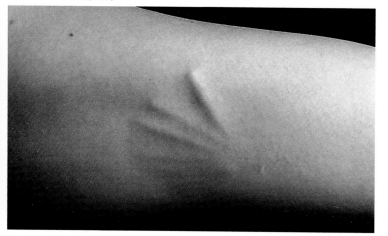

Fig. 47 Norplant.

Hormonal contraception (cont.)	*Postcoital contraception.* Two combined oral contraceptive pills containing 50 µg of estrogen are taken followed by a further two tablets 12 h later. They must be taken within 72 h of unprotected intercourse. This regimen causes nausea in up to 30% of takers. The overall failure rate is roughly 2%.
Intrauterine contraceptive devices	The IUCD (Fig. 48) is placed in the uterus by a physician using a sterile technique. It acts by altering/inhibiting sperm migration and ovum transport. The sterile inflammatory response to the presence of a foreign body inhibits implantation of the blastocyst. It is a safe, highly effective, and reversible form of contraception, but it must be fitted by a physician and requires follow-up care. An IUCD should not be fitted in women who have had pelvic inflammatory disease or if there is an intrauterine pregnancy or uterine abnormality. It can be used as a method of postcoital contraception. To be effective, it must be fitted within 5 days of unprotected intercourse.
Progesterone-releasing intra-uterine (IUS)	Progestogens are released into the uterine cavity and prevent proliferation and cause thickening of the cervical mucus. The devices also reduce menstrual blood loss and dysmenorrhea. They are one of the most effective reversible methods of contraception.
Sterilization	Female methods of sterilization involve the blockage of the fallopian tubes. This can be achieved by excision or occlusion with clips (Fig. 49) or rings or by diathermy via the laparoscope or a minilaparotomy. It is highly effective and should be considered irreversible. The failure rate is about 0.1%.
	Male sterilization is a good alternative to female sterilization and should be discussed with couples presenting to the gynecology clinic requesting sterilization.

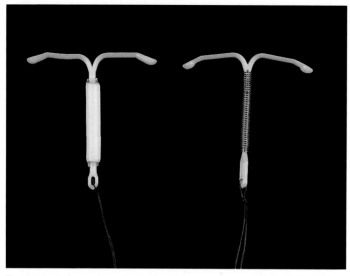

Fig. 48 Intrauterine contraceptive devices: (left) progestogen-containing IUS; (right) Nova T IUCD.

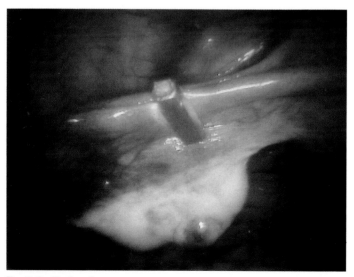

Fig. 49 Sterilization clip.

Miscarriage

Definition

A spontaneous loss of pregnancy before 24 weeks.

Incidence

15–25% of all pregnancies end in miscarriage.

Classification

Miscarriage can be classified as follows (Fig. 50):
- *Threatened abortion*: fetus is still viable, and the cervical os is closed.
- *Inevitable abortion*: fetus may still be alive but the cervical os is open.
- *Incomplete abortion*: some products of conception have been expelled already.
- *Complete abortion*: fetus and placental tissue have all been expelled.
- *Missed abortion*: the pregnancy has succumbed but has not been expelled (Fig. 51, p. 38).

Etiology

The majority of miscarriages are due to chromosomal defects. If they are in the first trimester, it is not worth investigating women who miscarry—unless they have had three consecutive spontaneous miscarriages. The causes can be:
- abnormal conceptus (chromosomal or structural)
- immunologic
- uterine abnormality
- cervical incompetence
- endocrine
- maternal disease (including systemic lupus erythematosus)
- infection
- toxins and cytotoxic drugs
- trauma

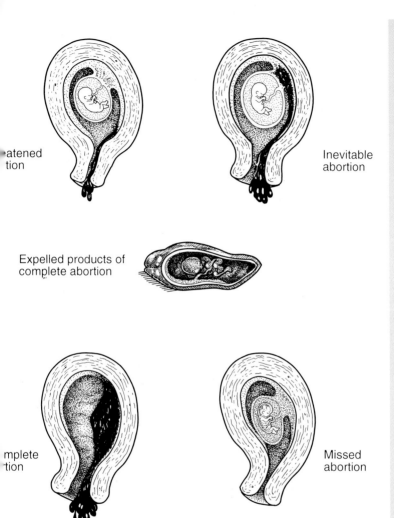

atened
tion

Inevitable
abortion

Expelled products of
complete abortion

mplete
tion

Missed
abortion

Fig. 50 Diagrammatic representation of types of miscarriage.

Clinical features of miscarriage	Patients will present with amenorrhea followed by vaginal bleeding. Pain may be present. The symptoms of pregnancy may have disappeared. On examination, there may be lower abdominal tenderness. The bleeding may vary from spotting to heavy bleeding. The uterine size may be smaller than dates (if products have been expelled), the same size, or larger than dates (if bleeding has occurred into the uterine cavity). The cervix may be closed or open, depending on the stage of the miscarriage.
Differential diagnosis	• Ectopic pregnancy. • Hydatidiform mole. • Dysfunctional uterine bleeding.
Investigation	If the cervical os is open, the pregnancy will not continue and no further investigations are needed. If the os is closed, an ultrasound scan will determine whether a viable fetus is present in the uterine cavity (Fig. 51).
Management	There is no proven treatment for a threatened abortion. Inevitable, incomplete, complete, and missed abortions all require evacuation of the uterus (Fig. 52).

Recurrent miscarriage

There is increasing evidence that women who recurrently miscarry may have anticardiolipin and antiphospholipid antibodies (antiphospholipid antibody syndrome). Women who have three or more miscarriages should be referred to a specialist unit where this can be investigated. Women with antiphospholipid antibodies syndrome also appear to be at risk of later pregnancy problems including preeclampsia and intrauterine growth retardation. The treatment may include heparin and the use of low-dose aspirin from as soon as a viable pregnancy is diagnosed.

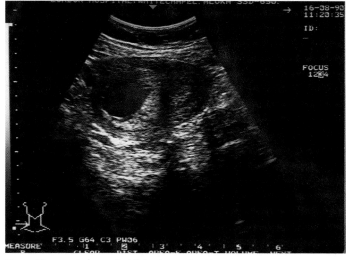

Fig. 51 Ultrasound picture of a blighted ovum in a bicornuate uterus.

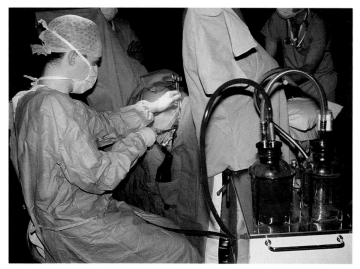

Fig. 52 Surgical evacuation of the uterus.

Ectopic pregnancy: diagnosis

Definition

The implantation of a pregnancy outside the uterine cavity (usually in the ampullary part of the fallopian tube).

Etiology

Any factor that will decrease embryo transport along the tube can lead to an ectopic pregnancy. The most common cause is previous pelvic infection.

Pathophysiology

The fertilized ovum is delayed in its transport along the tube and implants on the tubal mucosa. Intratubal or intraperitoneal bleeding occurs as a result of erosion and distension of the tubal wall (Fig. 53). The uterine endometrium undergoes decidualization in response to the hormonal stimulus of the trophoblast.

Symptoms

Classically, the patient will have had amenorrhea followed by irregular spotting or vaginal bleeding and unilateral pain (may be bilateral).

Signs

These will vary depending on whether tubal rupture has occurred. If tubal rupture has occurred, the patient may be in shock.

The abdominal signs can vary from unilateral lower abdominal tenderness with rebound to a rigid abdomen with guarding. Vaginally, there is usually cervical excitation and unilateral tenderness, and a mass may be felt on one side.

Differential diagnosis

- Miscarriage.
- Pelvic infection.

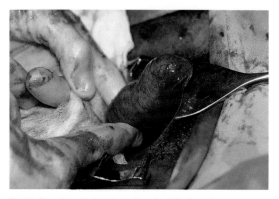

Fig. 53 Ectopic gestation distending the fallopian tube.

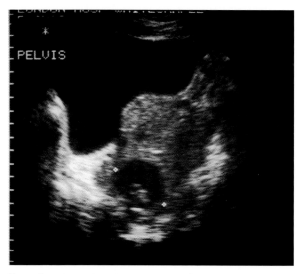

Fig. 54 Gestation sac lateral to the uterus, which is indenting the bladder.

Ectopic pregnancy: Management

Investigations for ectopic pregnancy

Pregnancy test: should be positive if modern HCG assay is used.

Ultrasound scan: may be useful if an intrauterine pregnancy is demonstrated. Occasionally, the ectopic pregnancy can be seen outside the uterine cavity (Fig. 54, p. 40), and free fluid can be seen in the pouch of Douglas.

Blood sampling: for complete blood count (CBC) and cross-matching.

Laparoscopy: should be performed if there is a suspicion of an ectopic pregnancy; the fallopian tube may appear distended or filled with blood (Fig. 55). Laparoscopic surgical techniques including linear salpingotomy, partial or total salpingectomy are very successful treatments for ectopic pregnancy, often avoiding the need for a laparotomy.

Laparotomy: should be considered if the patient is in shock due to a ruptured ectopic pregnancy or any situation that cannot be safely dealt with laparoscopically.

Treatment

Resuscitation if needed. Surgery should be conservative as above. Occasionally, a tubal abortion may have occurred, and the fetus may be free in the peritoneal cavity (Fig. 56).

Prognosis

Only one-third of women will proceed to have a successful term baby. About 10% will have a further ectopic pregnancy.

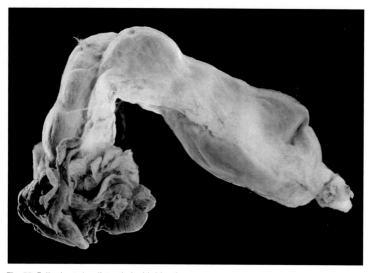

Fig. 55 Fallopian tube distended with blood.

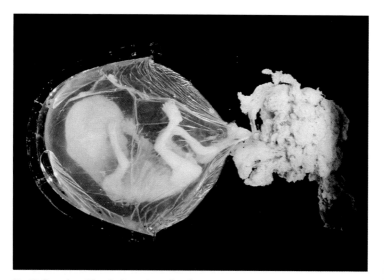

Fig. 56 Fetus found free in the peritoneal cavity.

Trophoblastic disease

Definition

Hydatidiform mole is a benign tumor of trophoblast.

Incidence

Varies geographically, with a higher incidence in Asiatic countries than in the West.

Etiology

Unknown.

Classification

Complete mole: no fetus is present, and the chromosomal complement is totally paternal. There are 46 chromosomes.

Partial mole: fetus is present. There are 69 chromosomes, and the extra set is of paternal origin.

Invasive mole: may penetrate the uterus and/or metastasize to the lungs.

Clinical features

The symptoms are usually irregular bleeding in the first trimester of pregnancy. The uterus may be larger than dates, and the fetal heart is usually absent. Preeclampsia may develop early, and theca lutein cysts may be palpable.

Investigations

Ultrasound will demonstrate a "snowstorm" appearance, and the fetus will not be seen (Fig. 57). Beta HCG level is very high. A chest radiograph should be done to exclude pulmonary metastases.

Management

Suction evacuation of the hydropic vesicles (Fig. 58). If uterine size is too large, extra-amniotic prostaglandins are used. Hysterectomy may be done in the older woman. It is essential to follow all women to ensure that the beta HCG levels disappear. Pregnancy should be discouraged for at least 12 months.

Prognosis

One in 30 moles develops into choriocarcinoma—a malignant tumor of trophoblastic tissue. Chemotherapy is the mainstay of treatment, and close follow-up is essential.

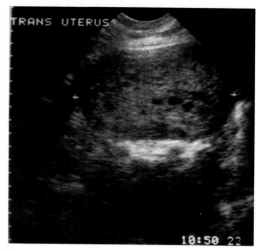

Fig. 57 Ultrasound picture of hydatidiform mole.

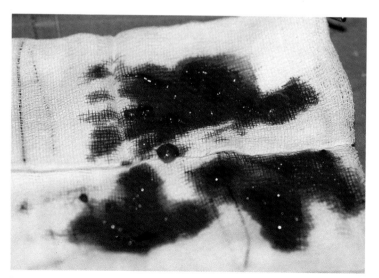

Fig. 58 Hydropic vesicles of hydatidiform mole.

7 / Therapeutic abortion

Definition	Medical or surgical termination of pregnancy prior to viability. The actual gestational age at which this occurs depends on the state in which the abortion is performed.
Classification	Terminations can be performed for fetal or maternal reasons. Most are performed because the continuation of the pregnancy will cause risk to the physical or mental health of the woman.
Investigations	If gestation is in doubt, an ultrasound scan should be performed. Complete blood count, blood group, rhesus status, and hemoglobin electrophoresis should be undertaken if indicated.
Management	Counseling is essential in pregnancy termination. The method of termination will depend on the gestation.

Progesterone antagonists.   These are not yet available in the United States for the termination of pregnancy, although Planned Parenthood does have the patent.

Dilation and evacuation (D&E).   The cervix is dilated by using Laminaria or Dilapan, and then the uterine contents are removed. D&E is a term reserved for termination beyond 14 week's, gestation. Before 14 weeks, the termination is called a suction D&C.

Prostaglandins.   Labor is induced with prostaglandins after 14 weeks' gestation. They can be administered as vaginal pessaries, intra-amniotically or extra-amniotically. The procedure is not followed by an evacuation of the uterus in the United States in 95% of cases, but D&Cs are performed on a symptomatic basis only.

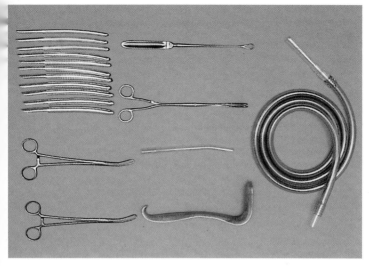

Fig. 59 Instruments used for suction termination of pregnancy.

Lower genital tract infections I

The most common manifestations are vaginal discharge and vulvovaginitis.

Etiology

Candida (thrush)

Most cases are due to *Candida albicians* (a yeast-like fungus). Yeasts may be present in the vagina without causing symptoms. *Candida* is not necessarily sexually transmitted; it can spread from the anus to the vulva and vagina. Once established, however, it can be transmitted sexually even by an asymptomatic partner.

Clinical features

Yeasts are the most common cause of vaginitis and vaginal discharge. The discharge is characteristically white, particulate, nonoffensive, and irritant. The vulva may appear red and edematous and/or covered in white discharge (Fig. 60). In the vagina, white discharge (the texture of cottage cheese) adheres to the vaginal walls (Fig. 61). Yeasts can be identified by microscopy and Gram staining of a high vaginal swab and by culture in the appropriate medium. Yeast is identified in vaginal discharges in the KOH test, which is a bedside slide with a drop of saline and a drop of KOH.

Management

Treatment includes topical antifungal agents, pessaries, and creams. Severe cases may require systemic therapy with oral antifungal agents (e.g., fluconazole).

Etiology

Trichomonas vaginalis (TV)

TV is a flagellate parasite found in the vagina, the urethra (of both men and women), and the upper genital tract. It is the second most common cause of vaginal discharge. It is sexually acquired and is often found in association with gonorrhea. The vaginal discharge is thin, yellow, offensive, and irritant, often appearing frothy and causing reddening of the vaginal mucosa and the cervix (Fig. 62, p. 50). The organism is identified by microscopy of a high vaginal sample mixed with a drop of saline.

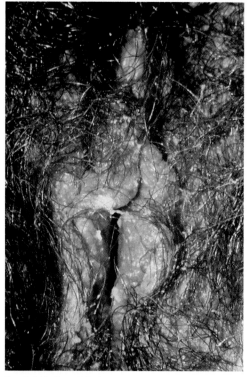

Fig. 60 Vulval candidiasis.

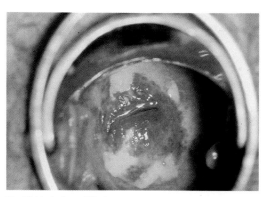

Fig. 61 Vaginal candidiasis.

Lower genital tract infections II

Bacterial vaginosis

This is characterized by an offensive vaginal discharge that gives a positive amine test, has a pH >5, and "clue cells" seen on microscopy of a Gram-stained smear. The cause is a mixed infection with *Gardnerella vaginalis* and anaerobic organisms including *Bacteroides* species and *Peptostreptococci*.

Treatment is with oral metronidazole or clindamycin cream.

Other causes of vaginal discharge include increased but normal vaginal secretion (e.g., at ovulation, during sexual excitement, or during pregnancy) and abnormal discharge due to chemical irritants, foreign bodies, or degenerative conditions.

Description

Warts (human papilloma virus: HPV)

Warts are caused by HPV. They can be flat and undetectable to the naked eye or large exophytic lesions. The cervix (Fig. 63) and vaginal and vulval surfaces (Fig. 64) are all susceptible to infection. HPV has been strongly implicated as a causative factor in cervical neoplasia. The incubation period varies from 3 weeks to 8 months. It may present as painless slow-growing vulvovaginal lumps. The differential diagnoses include molluscum contagiosum (caused by a pox virus), condylomata lata (lesions of secondary syphilis), and other skin tags, nevi, or sebaceous cysts.

Management

The following treatments are available: podophyllin (a cytotoxic agent), trichloracetic acid, laser vaporization, electrocautery, cryocautery, and excision. The last three are reserved for resistant and extensive warts. Barrier contraception is advised.

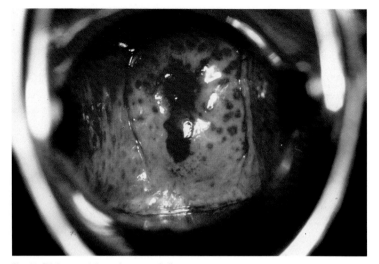

Fig. 62 Trichomonal "strawberry cervix."

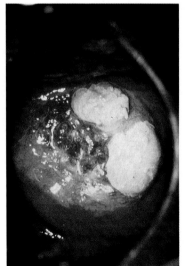

Fig. 63 Cervical warts.

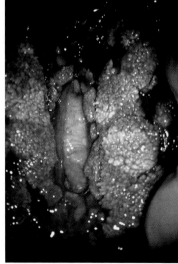

Fig. 64 Florid vulval warts.

Lower genital tract infections III

Etiology

Herpes simplex virus (HSV)

Genital and anal herpes are usually caused by type II HSV, but type I HSV (usually responsible for oral cold sores) can also be a cause of genital infection.

Clinical features

A primary infection may present with prodromal discomfort, followed by the appearance of vesicles (Fig. 65), ulceration, inguinal lymphadenopathy together with malaise, fever, and possibly urinary retention. In women, the vesicles are usually situated on the vulva (Fig. 66), vagina, and cervix. The lesions of a primary infection may take several weeks to heal, and secondary infection is common. Recurrence of HSV infection is common, as the virus lies dormant in the posterior nerve root ganglia between recurrences. Recurrent infection is less florid. Diagnosis is made on clinical examination and confirmed by viral cultures from the ulcers.

Management

Acyclovir can be used to reduce symptoms and virus shedding times in a primary attack. It does not prevent recurrences except during continuous treatment.

Complications

Primary infection can give rise to systemic complications, including hepatitis, myelitis, encephalitis, and meningitis. A primary infection in early pregnancy may cause abortion. Infection near term may be transmitted to the baby during delivery, leading to a high mortality rate and a high rate of neurologic complications in the survivors. Primary infection or active recurrent disease at term is an indication for delivery by cesarean section before rupture of the membranes.

Other pathogens

Chlamydia trachomatis and *Neisseria gonorrhoeae* infect the cervix and urethra. They are usually asymptomatic in the absence of spread to the upper genital tract.

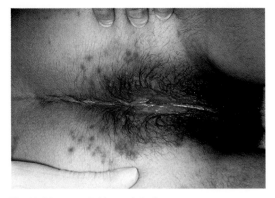

Fig. 65 Primary genital herpes infection.

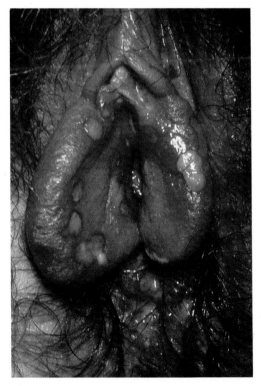

Fig. 66 Vulval herpes infection.

Pelvic inflammatory disease (PID)

Definition

An infection of the endometrium, fallopian tubes, and/or contiguous structures caused by the ascent of microorganisms from the lower genital tract.

Incidence

Most women who develop PID are younger than 25 years of age.

Etiology

The majority of cases of PID in young women are associated with sexually transmitted bacteria (e.g., *Chlamydia trachomatis* and *Neisseria gonorrhoeae*). These bacteria may initiate the process and then be replaced by opportunistic bacteria including streptococci and Bacteroides.

Clinical features

There is a spectrum of presentation from silent infection to florid symptoms and signs (i.e., pelvic pain, dyspareunia, fever, vaginal discharge, pyrexia, pelvic peritonism, cervical excitation, and possibly, a pelvic mass). Right upper-quadrant pain may be due to perihepatitis (Fig. 67). It complicates up to 15% of cases of chlamydial PID. Laparoscopic evidence of PID (Fig. 68) is seen in only 65% of suspected cases.

Differential diagnoses

These include acute appendicitis, endometriosis, ectopic pregnancy, ovarian cyst accident, and inflammatory bowel conditions.

Management

A combination of antibiotics active against all likely causative organisms, along with adequate analgesia, is required. In severe cases, hospital admission may be necessary. Surgery is appropriate if the condition fails to improve or deteriorates with conservative management. All women with PID and their partners should be referred to a genitourinary medicine clinic, screened for sexually transmitted infections, and treated appropriately to avoid reinfection.

Complications

Infertility follows in 15–20% of cases. There is a 7–10-fold increased risk of an ectopic pregnancy, and chronic pelvic pain is suffered by roughly 20% of women after PID.

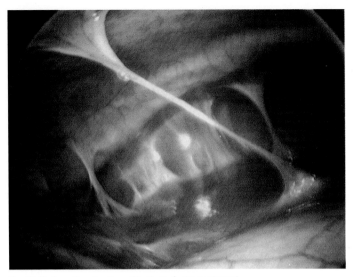

Fig. 67 Perihepatic adhesions (Fitz-Hugh–Curtis syndrome).

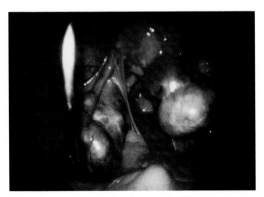

Fig. 68 Bilateral tubo-ovarian abscesses in PID.

HIV infection

Incidence and etiology

HIV (human immunodeficiency virus) is most prevalent in North and South America, sub-Saharan Africa, and western Europe. The age and sex distribution varies widely.

Mode of transmission

Sexual. Heterosexual intercourse is the most common mode of transmission/acquisition world-wide. In Europe and North America, women are accounting for an increasing proportion of new cases.

Parenteral. Spread is from blood and blood products, before screening and heat treatment were introduced in 1985, and from sharing infected needles.

Transmission from mother to fetus. From 11 to 30% of children born to HIV antibody-positive women will be infected (i.e., have antibodies persisting for greater than 18 months or develop clinical and or immunologic manifestations of HIV at an earlier stage). Maternal health is an important factor in transmission of infection to the fetus. Of those infants who acquire HIV from their mothers, about 25% will develop acquired immunodeficiency syndrome (AIDS) in the first year of life.

Clinical features

AIDS is defined as an illness caused by HIV and characterized by one or more "indicator" diseases, which include candidiasis of the gastrointestinal (Fig. 69) and respiratory tract, cryptosporidiosis, *Pneumocystis carinii* pneumonia (Fig. 70), and toxoplasmosis of the brain (Fig. 71). Kaposi's sarcoma (Fig. 72) is rare in women; otherwise, the spectrum of disease seen in men and women is similar.

Women and HIV

Important issues for women with HIV concern choice of contraception and wishes regarding pregnancy. There is no evidence that pregnancy accelerates the progress to AIDS. It has been suggested that the combined oral contraceptive pill may increase the risk of transmission and that an IUCD may put women with HIV at increased risk of pelvic inflammatory disease.

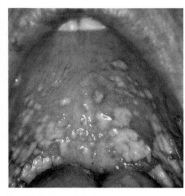

Fig. 69 Oral candidiasis.

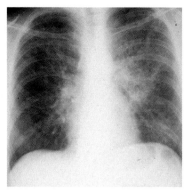

Fig. 70 *Pneumocystis carinii* pneumonia.

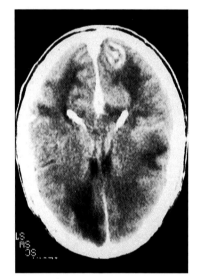

Fig. 71 Cerebral toxoplasmosis.

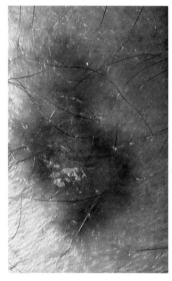

Fig. 72 Kaposi's sarcoma.

9 / Endometriosis

Diagnosis

Definition

Endometriosis is a benign process characterized by the presence and proliferation of endometrial tissue in sites outside the uterine cavity.

Incidence

It is seen in up to 10% of premenopausal white women and 30% of women presenting with infertility. The use of the oral contraceptive pill reduces the incidence of endometriosis.

Etiology

A number of theories regarding the pathogenesis of endometriosis exist, but no single theory will explain all cases. The condition may therefore result from a combination of the following:

- *Retrograde menstruation:* the passage of endometrial tissue along the fallopian tubes during menstruation with implantation in the peritoneal cavity.
- *Lymphatic or vascular spread:* endometrial tissue embolizing to distant sites.
- *Metaplasia of coelomic epithelium:* the repeated inflammatory insult from menstrual blood in the peritoneal cavity may lead to redifferentiation of the peritoneal tissue and the development of viable endometrial tissue.

Pathology

A noninfectious process of inflammation, fibrosis, and adhesion formation. The gross appearance is of black spots ("powder burns") (Fig. 73), commonly on the ovaries, uterosacral ligaments (Fig. 74), and pouch of Douglas. Adhesion formation and distortion of normal anatomy may be a feature in severe disease (Fig. 75). If the ovaries are involved, "chocolate cysts" may form. Unusual sites for endometriosis include the umbilicus, laparotomy scars, episiotomy scars, cervix, bowel, bladder, lung, thigh, and vulva.

Clinical features

These include pain, which may be cyclical, dyspareunia, backache, and secondary dysmenorrhea. Rarely, there may be hematuria or rectal bleeding if the bladder or bowel are involved. Endometriosis may also be symptomless.

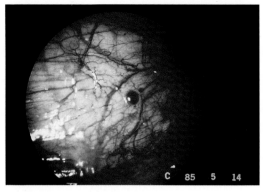

Fig. 73 Endometriotic deposit.

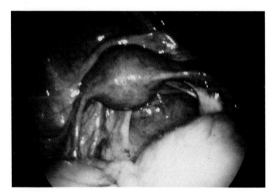

Fig. 74 Laparoscopy showing minimal endometriosis on left.

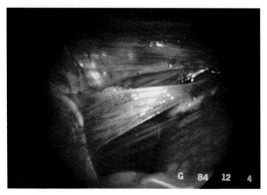

Fig. 75 Adhesions secondary to endometriosis.

Management

Examination

A thorough clinical examination is essential and may reveal localized endometrial deposits (e.g., cervical endometriosis) (Fig. 76).

Investigations

The definitive diagnosis is made by laparoscopy or laparotomy (Fig. 77). If hematuria or rectal bleeding are features, cystoscopy, sigmoidoscopy, and barium enema would be necessary.

Management

Symptomatic disease can be treated medically or surgically.

Medical treatment
Medical treatment is based on the observation that endometriosis improves in pregnancy. The use of the oral contraceptive pill, without breaks for withdrawal bleeds, for up to 9 months mimics pregnancy and is associated with symptomatic improvement. Progestogens (e.g., medroxyprogesterone acetate) also suppress ovulation and give relief from symptoms. Danazol (a testosterone derivative) is the most commonly used treatment. It creates a high-androgen, low-estrogen environment that does not support the growth of endometrium. Gestrinone acts similarly to Danazol and has the advantage of being taken twice weekly as opposed to twice daily. GnRH analogs given intranasally or subcutaneously suppress ovulation at the hypothalamus.

Many medical treatments are effective in the treatment of endometriosis, but unfortunately the condition can relapse. Side effects arise with all medications: breakthrough bleeding on the oral contraceptive pill; bloating and premenstrual syndrome-like symptoms with progestogen; androgenic side effects with Danazol; and hypoestrogenic effects such as hot flushes and bone loss with GnRH analogs. Medical treatment must be tailored to the individual patient.

Surgical treatment
Surgical approaches can be through the laparoscope (diathermy or laser ablation and division of adhesions) or by laparotomy to restore pelvic anatomy or remove the uterus and ovaries.

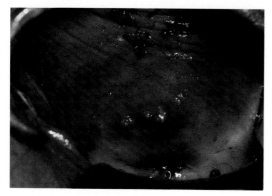

Fig. 76 Cervical endometriosis.

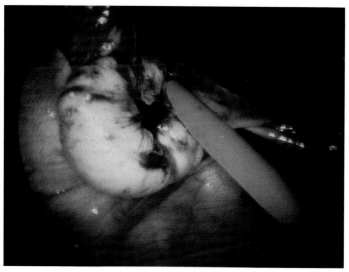

Fig. 77 Laparoscopic division of endometriotic adhesion.

Definition

Failure to conceive after 12 months of regular unprotected intercourse. One in six couples is affected.

Etiology

Three main causes of infertility: poor semen quality, tubal disorders, and ovulatory disorders. Other rarer causes include mucus "hostility" and sperm antibodies, impotence, and retrograde ejaculation. This leaves a significant (10–20%) proportion with unexplained infertility, which includes psychological factors.

Clinical features

Significant clues to the etiology can be achieved by a thorough history from both partners. In the female, evidence of ovulation can be gained from regularity of menstrual cycle and associated symptoms (e.g., mittelschmerz pain, cervical mucus changes, and primary dysmenorrhea).

Tubal disorders are usually the result of scarring and adhesions secondary to infection (Figs. 78 and 79) or pelvic surgery (e.g., ovarian cystectomy). In addition, endometriosis may cause pelvic scarring. If the distal portion of the tube is blocked, a hydrosalpinx may develop (Fig. 80). Tubal damage should be suspected if there is a history of IUCD use, PID, pelvic surgery, or pelvic pain.

Examination may also reveal endocrinologic disorders (e.g., polycystic ovarian syndrome [PCOS], or the tissue atrophy of premature menopause) and physical signs of pelvic pathology (e.g., endometriotic scarring, ovarian cysts or fibroids).

In the male, history may reveal previous operations or infections. Stress and recent intercurrent illnesses may be associated with transitory reduced semen quality. Examination should include testicles, looking for varicosities or the absence of the vas deferens. Reduced testicular size and increased firmness due to fibrosis may indicate spermatogenic failure. A swollen epididymis may indicate a blockage of the vas.

Rarely, azoospermia may be due to hypogonadotrophic hypogonadism, indicated by lack of secondary sexual development. ➡

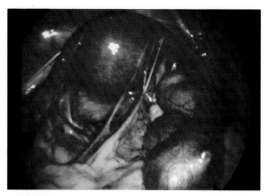

Fig. 78 Pelvic adhesions after PID.

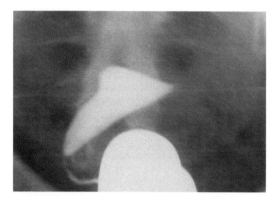

Fig. 79 Cornual blockage.

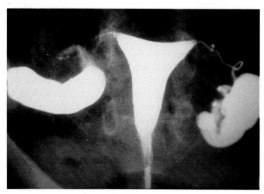

Fig. 80 Bilateral hydrosalpinges.

Defining the specific causes of infertility requires a proper history and examination and appropriate investigations as outlined below.

Male

For the male, a semen analysis on two occasions is the basic investigation. The World Health Organization criteria for a normal semen analysis is a sperm density of ≥ 20 million/ml with $\geq 50\%$ motility and $\geq 50\%$ normal sperm. The criteria are associated with a normal rate of conception. If the values are reduced, serum LH, FSH, and testosterone are indicated. High gonadotropins are indicative of testicular failure. Normal levels with reduced testosterone may indicate hypogonadotropic hypogonadism. There is rarely an indication for testicular biopsy.

Female

In the female, simple tests for ovulation should be undertaken (i.e., mid-luteal phase serum progesterone, basal body temperature charts [Fig. 81] for no more than two cycles). More sophisticated investigations include follicle monitoring with ultrasound (Fig. 82), serial LH measurements to detect the preovulatory LH surge, and laparoscopy in the luteal phase to confirm the presence of a corpus luteum.

Laparoscopy and dye instillations (Fig. 83) provide the optimum test of tubal patency or damage with additional benefit of visualization of the pelvis (i.e., ovaries [for the presence of corpus luteum], peritoneum to exclude endometriotic deposits, and the uterus to assess anatomic abnormality). Hysterosalpingography is used to assess tubal patency and also to reveal intrauterine problems (e.g., adhesions, fibroids, or anatomic abnormalities such as bicornuate uterus [Fig. 84]). Other investigations include a postcoital test, which assesses the capacity of sperm to remain motile in the cervical mucus, and tests for antisperm antibodies in both partners and in the husband's seminal plasma.

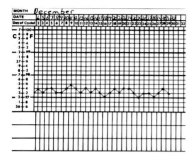

Fig. 81 Temperature chart showing an anovulatory pattern with absence of luteal phase rise.

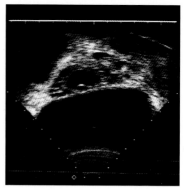

Fig. 82 Ultrasound image of a dominant follicle.

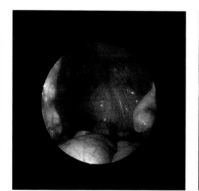

Fig. 83 Tubal patency as shown by presence of blue dye in the pelvis.

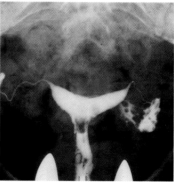

Fig. 84 Hysterosalpingogram of bicornuate uterus.

Male

Poor semen quality previously had little opportunity for improvement unless it was a transitory problem (e.g., stress or viral infection). The value of varicocele repair is unresolved. Hormonal treatments are unproven. With low counts, options that are now available include the preparation of a small volume of the best sperm to place within the uterus at ovulation (intrauterine insemination) or in vitro fertilization (IVF) with oocytes collected from the patient. Intracytoplasmic sperm injection (ICSI) has dramatically altered the treatment of severe male factor infertility. ICSI only requires low sperm numbers and can be used in the treatment of both obstructive and nonobstructive azoospermia. Antisperm antibodies have been successfully treated with steroids in the male. Donor semen remains the only option for many infertile men.

Female

Ovulatory disorders respond well to hormonal therapy (i.e., clomiphene or human menopausal gonadotropins). The latter requires close monitoring to avoid hyperstimulation or high-order multiple pregnancy. The damage can be dealt with by tubal surgery (Fig. 85) in selected cases, but the results rarely exceed 30%.

Bypassing the tube with IVF is successful in 15–20% of cycles. This involves ovarian stimulation to produce multiple follicles, the aspiration of the oocytes from these follicles, the IVF with partner's semen, and transfer to the uterus 48 h after fertilization.

Assisted conception techniques including IVF and gamete intrafallopian transfer (Fig. 86) are also applicable when mucus hostility is a possible cause or when no cause is found (e.g., unexplained infertility). Success rates in these groups are between 25–30%.

Complications

The major complication of infertility other than those associated with drugs and surgical intervention is the psychological trauma of being unable to conceive. Significant morbidity is present in many couples who require counseling and support to enable them to come to terms with childlessness.

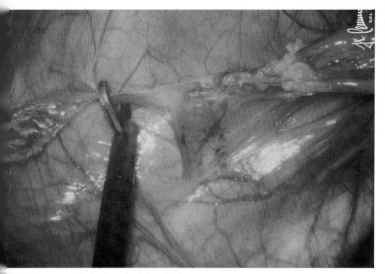

Fig. 85 Laparoscopic freeing of pelvic adhesions.

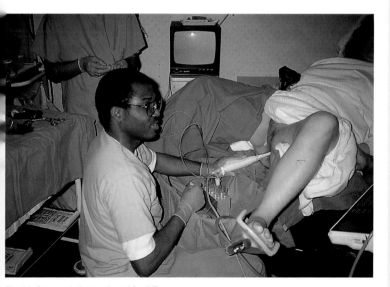

Fig. 86 Oocytes being aspirated for IVF.

11 / Polycystic ovarian syndrome

Definition

PCOS is a syndrome that consists of oligoamenorrhea, hirsutism (Figs. 87 and 88), obesity, and infertility; it is associated with disordered pituitary gonadotropin secretion and ovarian steroid production. It is a spectrum of disease as normally cycling women may have polycystic ovaries and yet none of the features above.

Incidence

Depending on the criteria used (clinical or ultrasound), the incidence varies from 5–30% of the female population. Among amenorrheic women, 30–40% probably have PCOS. Among hirsute women that incidence rises to 50–70%.

Etiology

The cause of PCOS is uncertain. There are two main hypotheses:
- ovarian enzyme abnormality resulting in abnormal steroid production
- disordered feedback mechanisms acting on the pituitary, resulting in abnormal gonadotropin secretion with secondary ovarian dysfunction

A small proportion of PCOS cases have been shown to be familial and due to ovarian enzyme abnormalities. The net result is an increased LH secretion, anovulation, and increased ovarian androgen production.

Pathology

The classic polycystic ovary is increased in size due to:
- increased stromal tissue
- multiple cystic ovaries, 2–4 mm in diameter, distributed around the periphery of the ovary (pearl nodi; Fig. 89).

Clinical features

Obesity is usually present from childhood, whereas hirsutism usually appears at puberty, affecting the face, chest, and abdomen. Oligoamenorrhea is present from puberty, often with episodes of secondary amenorrhea. Infertility is usually primary. ➡

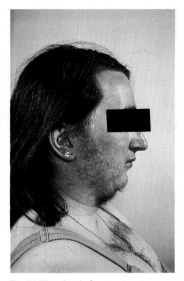

Fig. 87 Hirsutism before treatment.

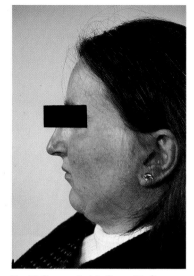

Fig. 88 Same patient in Figure 87 after hormone treatment.

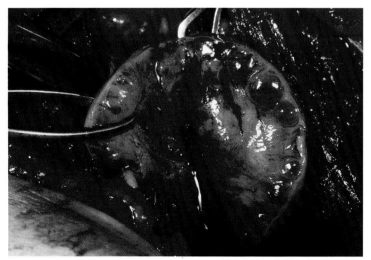

Fig. 89 Cut surface of polycystic ovary.

Differential diagnosis	Increased adrenal androgen production could also mean: • Cushing syndrome • adrenal hyperplasia • adrenal carcinoma Hirsutism could also be familial or due to drugs, whereas other causes of secondary amenorrhea include hyperprolactinemia. Other causes of infertility can be found on page 61.
Investigation	*Biochemical:* serum LH, FSH, prolactin, testosterone dehydroepiandrosterone sulfate, androstenedione). *Ultrasound:* ovaries and pelvis (Fig. 90) (laparoscopy/ovarian biopsy).
Management	*Hirsutism:* management includes: • cosmetic treatments (cream, waxing, and electrolysis) • oral contraceptive pill with low androgenic progestogen • antiandrogens (cyproterone acetate [Fig. 88, p. 68] and spironolactone) *Obesity* is treated with diet. *Oligoamenorrhea/amenorrhea:* treatment includes: • oral contraceptive pill to produce regular withdrawal bleeds • clomiphene (will produce regular cycles in 50% but will also induce ovulation) *Infertility:* induction of ovulation with clomiphene is successful in 70–80% of women with PCOS, with pregnancy rates equivalent to regularly ovulating women. If not successful, human menopausal gonadotropin, with or without pituitary down-regulation using luteinizing hormone releasing hormone analogs, is usually effective. This latter regime can result in severe ovarian hyperstimulation (Fig. 91).
Complications	This group of obese anovulatory women are more likely to develop endometrial hyperplasia and adenocarcinoma in later life. Regular shedding of the endometrium induced by progestogens or oral contraceptive pill seems a logical, although unproven, prophylaxis.

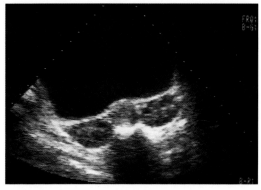

Fig. 90 Ultrasound showing polycystic ovaries.

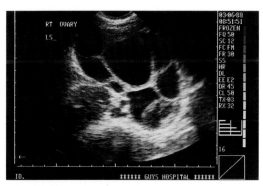

Fig. 91 Hyperstimulation in a polycystic ovary as seen by ultrasound.

Pruritus vulvae

Etiology

Vulval irritation can occur at any age, and the causes are numerous. The most common are infection, estrogen deficiency, and vulval dystrophies in the older woman.

Pathology

The most common infective agent is *Candida*. Non-infectious causes include lichen sclerosus, Paget's disease, and vulval intraepithelial neoplasia (VIN). Paget's disease of the vulva usually presents in the elderly (Fig. 92). VIN is a precursor to invasive carcinoma.

Clinical features

Irritation and itchiness of the vulva are present. On examination, there may be evidence of excoriation, discoloration (Fig. 93), and thickening or thinning of the vulval skin.

Bartholin's glands

These are paired structures that lie deep to the posterior introitus. They can become infected and present as a large tender swollen abscess. This is treated by a stab incision and insertion of a WORD catheter. Cyst formation can also occur.

Urethral caruncle

The external urethral meatus protrudes (Fig. 94) and swells. It may bleed and may be very tender. Urethral caruncles are often associated with infection. If surgery is performed, the excised piece of tissue should be sent for histologic confirmation to exclude urethral carcinoma.

Condylomata acuminata

Venereal warts are common on the vulva (Fig. 95) or in the vagina. They can be treated by topical applications, local destructive methods, or surgery.

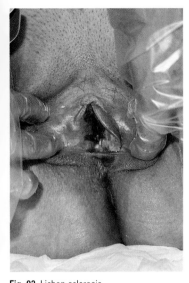

Fig. 92 Lichen sclerosis.

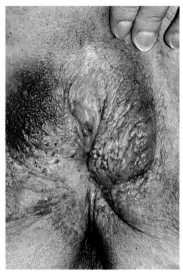

Fig. 93 Paget's disease of the vulva.

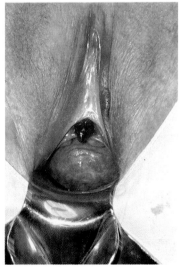

Fig. 94 Urethral caruncle with cystocoele.

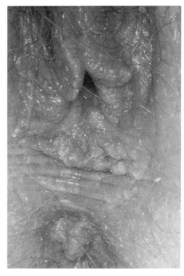

Fig. 95 Vulval warts.

Carcinoma of the vulva

Incidence

Vulval carcinoma is an uncommon disease confined to elderly women.

Etiology

The vulva is an ideal site for skin irritation—warm and moist, prone to friction, poor hygiene, and scratching.

Pathology

Carcinoma of the vulva (Fig. 96) is usually a slow-growing and well-differentiated squamous carcinoma. Most of the lymphatics drain directly to the superficial and deep inguinal nodes and then to the iliac chain.

Clinical features

The woman usually presents with a history of chronic vulval irritation. She may have delayed seeking advice owing to embarrassment. The lesion is usually an epitheliomatous ulcer but sometimes may be in a "cauliflower" form. The surrounding epithelium may show features of an underlying vulval dystrophy.

Management

All suspicious lesions must be biopsied. If vulval intraepithelial neoplasia is diagnosed, excision may be appropriate. Invasive carcinoma is best managed by radical vulvectomy, which consists of excision of the vulva (Figs. 97 and 98) and removal of the inguinal and femoral lymph nodes by using separate groin incisions for the lymphadenectomy as opposed to an en bloc removal as in Figure 99. This does not compromise the success of the operation and reduces morbidity associated with poor wound healing. Complications include lymphocoele formation at the groin as a consequence of node dissection, and these usually resolve with intermittent drainage. Lymphedema can be a chronic complication.

Complications

The morbidity and mortality from the operation are high, but the alternative is an unpleasant demise from a foul, fungating, and painful growth.

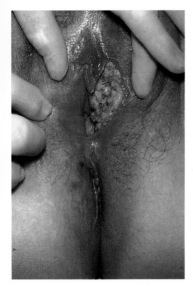

Fig. 96 Invasive carcinoma.

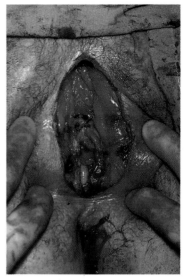

Fig. 97 Excision of the vulva.

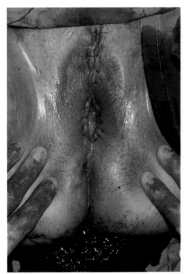

Fig. 98 Postoperative appearance.

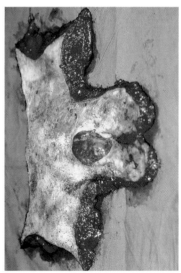

Fig. 99 Surgical specimen of vulval carcinoma.

13 / Benign, premalignant, and malignant conditions of the vaginal cervix

Normal cervix

The normal ectocervix is covered with stratified squamous epithelium. The endocervical canal is lined by columnar epithelium. The junction between these two types is known as the *squamocolumnar junction*.

The position of the squamocolumnar junction varies. Puberty, pregnancy, and the use of the oral contraceptive pill cause eversion of the canal, thereby displaying a greater area of columnar epithelium, which has a red appearance to the naked eye. This is termed *ectopy*. It is a normal physiologic response, and the term *erosion* should not be used in this context. The area medial to the squamocolumnar junction is called the *transformation zone*.

Benign conditions

Cervicitis

Certain bacteria preferentially infect columnar epithelium (e.g., *Chlamydia trachomatis* and *Neisseria gonorrhoeae*) giving rise to appearances described as cervicitis (Fig. 100).

Cervical fibroids

These may be pedunculated or within the body of the cervix (Fig. 101), perhaps growing to a size that fills the vagina.

Cervical polyps

These usually arise from the endocervix and are pedunculated with a covering of endocervical epithelium. They vary considerably in size and appear as bright red vascular growths (Fig. 102). Endocervical polyps may be symptomless or may present with irregular vaginal bleeding and/or postcoital bleeding. Treatment is by avulsion. If the base is broad, it may require ligation.

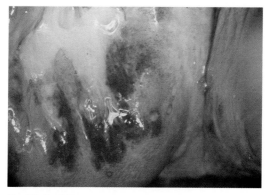

Fig. 100 Cervicitis.

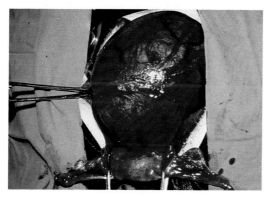

Fig. 101 Cervical fibroid at abdominal hysterectomy.

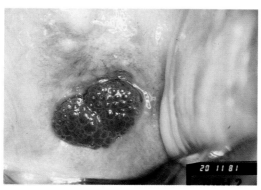

Fig. 102 Endocervical polyp. Colpophotograph.

Premalignant conditions: diagnosis

The transformation zone of the cervix normally undergoes metaplasia. However, it may, under certain circumstances, also become dysplastic.

Clinical features

Premalignant conditions of the cervix do not look abnormal to the naked eye. They are identified by cervical smear screening. The smear may demonstrate dyskaryotic cells (Fig. 103), graded as mild, moderate, or severe (Fig. 104), depending on the degree of atypia. A dyskaryotic cell is clearly recognizable as a squamous cell but displays some of the features of malignancy: the nucleus is enlarged, the chromatin is increased, and the nuclear borders are irregular.

Investigations

Women should have smears taken at 3-year intervals. If the smear is reported as showing mildly dyskaryotic cells, the smear should be repeated in 6 months. If these changes persist or worsen, referral for colposcopy is indicated. Women with one smear showing either moderate or severe dyskaryosis should be referred directly for colposcopy.

Colposcopy is used to identify the lesion giving rise to the dyskaryotic cells exfoliated by the cervical smear. Using acetic acid to stain the cervix, areas of immature metaplasia and dysplasia (Fig. 105) are seen as white ("acetowhite"). The density of this whiteness together with other features, including *punctation* (Fig. 106), *mosaicism* (Fig. 107, p. 80), and *atypical vessel formation*, suggest the degree of abnormality present. Punch biopsies are taken from these abnormal areas to make a histologic diagnosis.

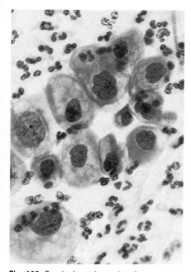

Fig. 103 Cervical cytology showing dyskaryosis.

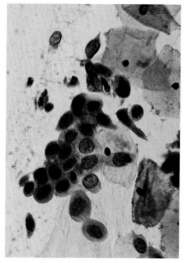

Fig. 104 Cervical cytology showing severe dyskaryosis.

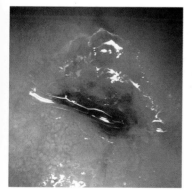

Fig. 105 Acetowhite changes.

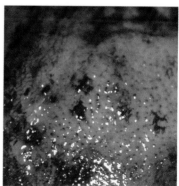

Fig. 106 Marked punctation.

Grading

The histologic findings are graded as CIN (cervical intraepithelial neoplasia) I, II, and III, depending on the degree of dysplasia. *Dysplasia* is a histologic term used to describe a lesion in which part of the thickness of the epithelium is replaced by atypical cells (Fig. 108).

If untreated, CIN may progress to cervical cancer.

CIN I—the atypia is confined to the basal one-third of the epithelium.

CIN II—the basal two-thirds are involved and the changes are more marked.

CIN III—nuclear abnormalities are present throughout the whole thickness of the epithelium (Figs. 109 and 110).

Predisposing factors

These include young age at first intercourse, the level of sexual activity in women and their partners, prolonged use of the oral contraceptive, and cigarette smoking.

Management

Destruction of the whole transformation zone including all the areas of abnormal epithelium is undertaken by using laser, cold coagulation, electrocautery, diathermy loop excision, or cone biopsy. Biopsy is performed along with endocervical curettage in the United States. Cone biopsy is reserved for cases in which colposcopic visualization of the transformation zone is incomplete. It is associated with risks of hemorrhage, cervical stenosis, and cervical incompetence. Electrocautery and cone biopsy are performed under general anesthetic, whereas all the others can be performed under local anesthesia.

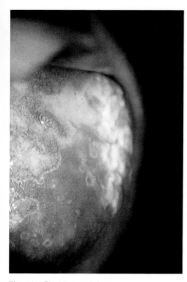

Fig. 107 Florid mosaicism.

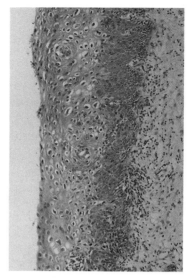

Fig. 108 Human papilloma virus and CIN.

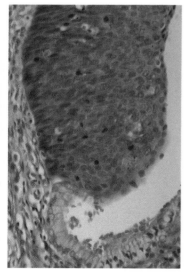

Fig. 109 CIN III and normal endocervix.

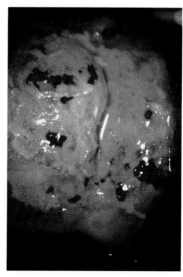

Fig. 110 Macroscopic view of CIN III.

Carcinoma of the cervix

Incidence

Despite a screening program aimed at the prevention of cervical cancer, the incidence is continuing to rise. For example, in England and Wales there are approximately 4,000 new cases reported each year. About 50% of these women will die from the disease within 5 years of diagnosis.

Etiology

Carcinoma of the cervix is more frequently seen in developing countries, and its incidence is higher in lower socioeconomic groups. Cancer of the cervix is essentially a sexually transmitted disease.

A number of factors may predispose to cervical cancer. Presently, the wart virus has the strongest association. Smoking may also have a role.

Staging

Cancer of the cervix is staged clinically. An examination under anesthesia is performed, combined with cervical biopsy, hysteroscopy and sampling, and cystoscopy.

Stage I
- Ia Microinvasive disease. Lesions with a depth of invasion through the basement membrane of <5 mm and with a horizontal spread of <7 mm (Fig. 111).
- Ib All other cases confined to the cervix (Fig. 112).

Stage II
The carcinoma extends beyond the cervix but has not extended onto the pelvic side wall. The carcinoma involves the vagina but not as far as the lower one-third.

Stage III
Carcinoma extends to the pelvic side wall. The lower one-third of the vagina may be involved. All cases with a hydronephrosis or a nonfunctioning kidney, unless they are known to be due to another cause.

Stage IV
Carcinoma has extended beyond the true pelvis or has clinically involved the mucosa of the bladder or rectum. ➡

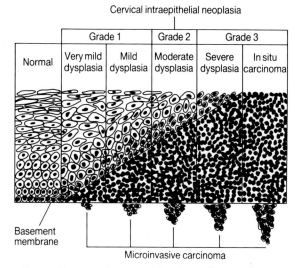

Fig. 111 Diagrammatic representation of premalignant and microinvasive disease (microinvasion is shown as crossing the basement membrane).

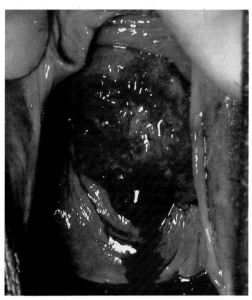

Fig. 112 Frank invasive carcinoma of the cervix.

Pathology	Up to 90% of cervical cancers are squamous cell tumors originating in the transformation zone. Adenocarcinomas account for the remainder of cases. Cervical cancer spreads by direct extension or via the lymphatics.
Clinical features	Patients may present with vaginal bleeding, particularly after intercourse. There may be vaginal discharge. Early lesions may be symptomless and are detected by screening.
Investigations	Once the diagnosis is confirmed histologically (Fig. 113), an examination under anesthesia is necessary for staging. Chest radiograph, intravenous pyelography, and routine biochemical and hematologic investigations are usually required. Computed tomographic scanning is helpful in advanced and recurrent disease.
Management	Hysterectomy is usually advised for microinvasive disease. Cone biopsy may be considered in a young woman desiring children. Stage Ib or IIa cervical cancer can be treated by either radiotherapy or radical Wertheim's hysterectomy (removal of the uterus, fallopian tubes, upper one-third of the vagina, parametrium, and pelvic lymph nodes). Wertheim's hysterectomy is the treatment of choice in younger women who wish to retain ovarian function and avoid vaginal stenosis and gastrointestinal side effects that may be caused by radiotherapy. The results of radiotherapy and radical surgery in early stage disease are similar, both having 5-year survival rates in excess of 80%. The finding of tumor in lymph nodes will halve this survival rate. Radiotherapy is commonly used in more advanced disease. The role of chemotherapy is under evaluation.
	Carcinoma of the vagina: rare and tends to occur mainly in the 6th and 7th decades. Presenting symptoms are vaginal bleeding or a purulent discharge. Treatment of the condition is determined by histology, staging, and the health of the patient. Surgery, radiotherapy, and a combination of both have been used.

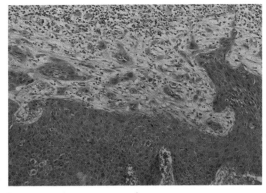

Fig. 113 Invasive squamous carcinoma.

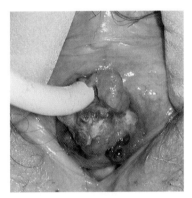

Fig. 114 Vaginal carcinoma.

Congenital anomalies

Congenital absence of the uterus is rare, and in such cases, a rudimentary vagina may be present. Congenital anomalies range from an arcuate uterus to a complete duplication of the uterus and cervix (Figs. 115 and 116).

Fibroids

Definition

Common smooth muscle tumors also known as leiomyomata. Etiology unknown.

Incidence

Fibroids occur in >20% of white women older than 30 years.

Classification

- *Subserous:* project from the peritoneal surface of the uterus.
- *Intramural:* lie within the uterine wall.
- *Submucous:* encroach on the uterine cavity.
- *Pedunculated:* can arise from subserous or submucous.

Pathology

Fibroids arise from smooth muscle cells during reproductive life and can increase in size in response to estrogen.

Clinical features

The majority of fibroids are symptomless. They may cause menorrhagia, abdominal distension, and pressure symptoms such as urinary frequency. Pain is unusual unless there is red degeneration or torsion of a pedunculated fibroid.

Abdominal examination may reveal a palpable mass arising from the pelvis. Pelvic examination will confirm this, and the outline may be irregular.

Investigations

These include ultrasonography, EUA, hysteroscopy, and D&C if abnormal bleeding.

Management of fibroids

Treatment can either be conservative or surgical (Fig. 117).

Complications

The poor vascularity of fibroids encourages degeneration (hyaline, cystic, red, sarcomatous), calcification (Fig. 118), and/or necrosis. Fibroids can also become infected, tort, and rarely metastasize.

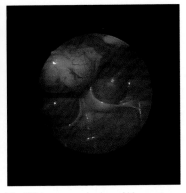

Fig. 115 Laparoscopic view of bicornuate uterus.

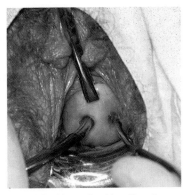

Fig. 116 Double cervix with a dilator in each os.

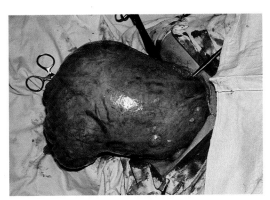

Fig. 117 Enlarged fibroid uterus—operative specimen.

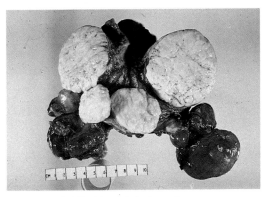

Fig. 118 Calcified fibroids—pathologic specimen.

Endometrial carcinoma

Classification

The majority of lesions are adenocarcinoma (Fig. 118, p. 86), and the staging is as follows:
Stage I—confined to the body of the uterus.
Stage II—involves the body and the cervix.
Stage III—extends beyond uterus but not beyond the true pelvis.
Stage IV—extends outside true pelvis or involves bladder or rectum.

Etiology

Endometrial carcinoma occurs in postmenopausal women and women who have had prolonged exposure to estrogen stimulation (i.e., nulliparous women, late menopause, obese women, and women with polycystic ovaries). Hyperplasia is a precursor.

Clinical features

Postmenopausal bleeding is the classic presentation for endometrial carcinoma and therefore requires investigation. It is rare in women younger than the age of 40, unless there are predisposing factors (e.g., PCO).

Investigations

Abdominal and pelvic examinations should be carried out in all cases. A cervical smear should be taken and endometrial sampling considered. Endometrial sampling can be performed in the outpatient clinic. Transvaginal ultrasound scanning may be helpful in identifying changes (>5 mm endometrial thickening is suspicious). Instilling fluid into the endometrial cavity at the time of transvaginal scanning may improve diagnostic accuracy. If outpatient sampling is not possible, then hysteroscopic assessment becomes necessary (Figs. 119 and 120).

Management

A total abdominal hysterectomy and bilateral salpingo-oophorectomy is performed during a staging operation that involves taking peritoneal washings and sampling enlarged pelvic and para-aortic nodes. Adjuvant radiotherapy is sometimes necessary to complete treatment for high-grade lesions and cancers that involve the outer half of the endometrium.

Progress

Factors influencing survival of endometrial carcinoma are age at diagnosis, stage of disease, pathologic type and degree of differentiation of the lesion, and the depth of myometrial invasion.

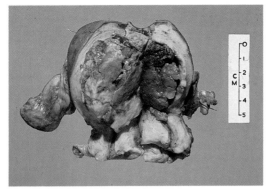

Fig. 119 Pathologic specimen of an endometrial cancer invading the endometrium.

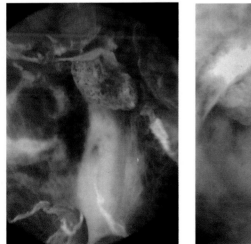 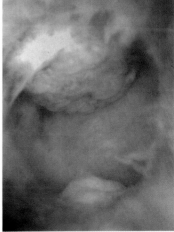

Fig. 120 Hysteroscopic view of endometrial carcinoma invading the endometrium.

15 / Benign and malignant conditions of the fallopian tubes

Introduction

The fimbriae of the fallopian tubes pick up the ovum after it is released from the follicle, and the cilia of the endosalpinx transport it to the site of fertilization. Sperm are transported by the cilia from the uterine end of the tube laterally to the site of fertilization.

Tubal infection

The tubes can become blocked by infection (or inflammation following trauma). The result of this can be tubal abscess or hydrosalpinx (Fig. 121).

Clinical features

Tubal infection may present with pain of an acute abdomen, especially if an abscess has formed. A hydrosalpinx may be symptomless.

Investigations

Laparoscopy is useful for inspection of the peritoneal aspect of the tubes. Exudate may be seen over the tubes, especially at the fimbriae. If the fimbriae are clubbed, this indicates chronic damage. Fresh and old adhesions may be seen. A hydrosalpinx will be visualized as a swollen tube but not actively infected. In the absence of acute infection, dye can be injected through the cervix. If there is no tubal blockage, filling of the tubes and free spill into the peritoneal cavity can be seen. Hysterosalpingography is a useful investigative technique.

Management

Acute infection should be treated appropriately. Infertility due to tubal damage can be treated by tubal surgery or in vitro fertilization to overcome tubal blockage.

Carcinoma of the fallopian tube

Primary carcinoma of the fallopian tube (Fig. 122) is rare; secondary disease from adjacent structures is more common. The symptoms are classically a watery, bloody vaginal discharge. On examination, an adnexal mass may be felt. The treatment is total abdominal hysterectomy and bilateral oophorectomy.

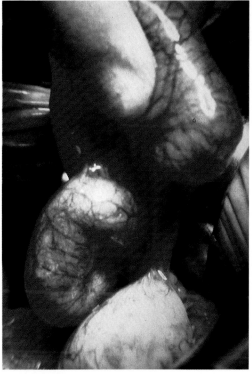

Fig. 121 Hydrosalpinx.

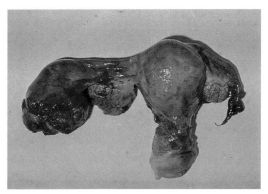

Fig. 122 Carcinoma of the fallopian tube.

Introduction

Ovarian cysts may be physiologic, benign (Fig. 123) or malignant tumors. Ovarian pathology may give rise to symptoms:

- when ovarian enlargement causes pressure on the bladder or rectum or abdominal distension
- if the ovary/cyst torts, bleeds, or ruptures
- should hormonal production be affected

Physiologic cysts (distension cysts)

Clinical types

Follicular cysts: due to enlargement of follicles that fail to rupture. They may be associated with anovulatory cycles, fertility drugs, and PCO. Usually symptomless and resolve spontaneously.

Corpus luteum cysts: can cause amenorrhea followed by heavy vaginal bleeding. Spontaneous resolution is the norm, but intra-abdominal bleeding may cause significant pain.

Endometriomas: result from invagination of endometrial deposits on the surface of the ovary.

Polycystic ovaries: enlarged (Fig. 124), with numerous small subcapsular follicular cysts.

Ovarian tumors—benign and malignant

Incidence

Benign tumors of the ovary are common. The incidence of ovarian cancer increases with age, with the peak incidence in the 60s.

Clinical features

Ovarian cancer is often either symptomless or associated with nonspecific symptoms such as dyspepsia. A malignant tumor should be suspected in older women, especially if it is fixed, bilateral, rapid-growing, or associated with ascites. A solid or a mixed cystic and solid appearance on ultrasound scanning is also suggestive. In advanced disease, there may be venous obstruction of the legs, pain, and palpable supraclavicular lymphadenopathy.

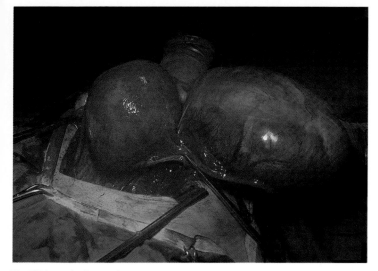

Fig. 123 Large benign ovarian cyst.

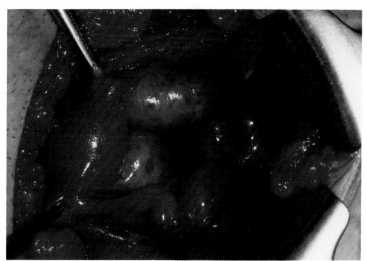

Fig. 124 "Kissing" polycystic ovaries.

Classification

Ovarian tumors can be derived from the following cell types:

- surface epithelium
- germ cells
- gonadal stroma

Secondary deposits from primary tumors of the breast, stomach, large bowel, and uterus may also occur in the ovaries (Krukenberg tumors; Fig. 125).

Tumors derived from surface epithelium

About 90% of ovarian tumors originate from the surface epithelium. These are further subdivided into:

- *serous* (e.g., serous cystadenoma [benign], serous cystadenocarcinoma [malignant, Fig. 126)
- *mucinous* (e.g., mucinous cystadenoma, mucinous cystadenocarcinoma)
- *endometrioid*
- *Brenner tumors*
- *clear cell tumors*

Epithelial ovarian tumors can be benign, of borderline malignancy, or frankly malignant. The malignant forms are collectively known as adenocarcinoma of the ovary.

Tumors derived from germ cells

The germ cells of the ovary are totipotent (i.e., can give rise to various types of tissues). Tumors of germ cells can contain a variety of tissues including teeth, bone, cartilage, muscle, thyroid, and nervous tissue. The most common germ cell tumor is the benign cystic teratoma (dermoid cyst, Fig. 127). These are the most common tumors in young women. They are bilateral in 10–20% of cases.

Tumors derived from gonadal stroma

Sex cord tumors are rare. Granulosa cell tumors and thecomas secrete estrogens and can therefore cause precocious puberty in premenarchal girls and endometrial hyperplasia and postmenopausal bleeding in older women. More than 50% of granulosa cell tumors are malignant; the vast majority of thecomas are benign. Sertoli–Leydig tumors may secrete androgens and can therefore cause progressive virilization.

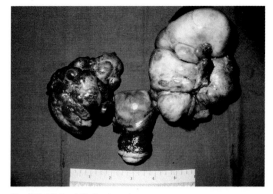

Fig. 125 Bilateral Krukenberg tumors.

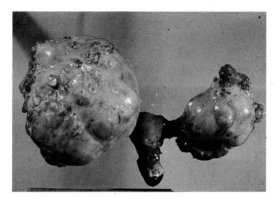

Fig. 126 Serous cystadenocarcinoma.

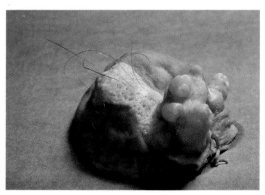

Fig. 127 Benign cystic teratoma.

Management

Benign tumors

Before embarking on surgery, the risk of malignancy must be assessed to prevent inexperienced surgeons encountering ovarian cancer (Figs. 128 and 129).

Ovarian cancer

An adequate preoperative assessment should be made, with a general examination including the breasts and lymph nodes. Laparotomy aims include adequate staging and removal of all visible tumor deposits (Figs. 130 and 131).

Staging requires thorough inspection of the whole abdominal cavity through a vertical incision. Peritoneal washings are taken, and the following are either removed or biopsied: parietal peritoneum, omentum, uterus and other ovary, bowel and mesentery, diaphragm, and pelvic and para-aortic lymph nodes.

Surgical measures

In early disease (i.e., stage I) total abdominal hysterectomy, bilateral salpingo-oophorectomy, omentectomy, and lymph node biopsy are necessary. In more advanced disease, the aim of surgery is to perform maximum debulking followed by chemotherapy.

Prognosis

The 5-year survival rates for primary ovarian cancer are as follows: Ia 85%, Ib–IIa 40%, IIb 25%, IIc–III 15%, IV < 5%. The prognosis has changed very little in the past 30 years because women continue to present late in the disease process.

Effective screening would be of value if it were possible to detect disease in its early stages, thereby enabling more effective treatment. Ultrasound scanning and various tumor markers (e.g., CA 125) are being evaluated but are as yet to be of proven value.

However, screening of women with a family history (i.e., two or more first-degree relatives with ovarian cancer) may be appropriate. This group of women only accounts for 5–10% of cases of ovarian cancer, but they have a lifetime risk of developing the diseases of 20–30%. Prophylactic oophorectomy may be appropriate for these women once they have completed childbearing.

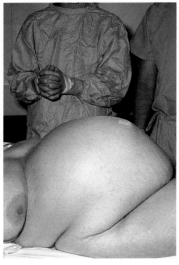

Fig. 128 Gross abdominal distension due to ovarian tumor.

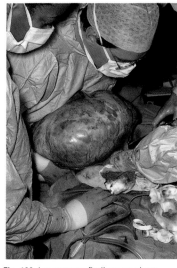

Fig. 129 Laparotomy findings on above.

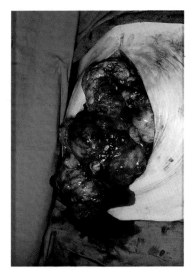

Fig. 130 Disseminated ovarian adenocarcinoma.

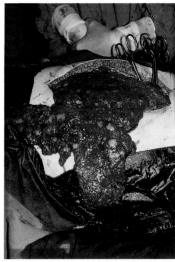

Fig. 131 Omental infiltration with ovarian adenocarcinoma.

Clinical features and pathology

Definition

The menopause is a woman's last menstrual period; the climacteric is the period of ovarian decline that includes the menopause.

Etiology

At the beginning of the climacteric, the remaining ovarian follicles become increasingly resistant to gonadotropin stimulation, and so more gonadotropins are produced in response to the decreasing estrogen levels.

Pathology

Atrophy occurs in all tissues that are sensitive to estrogen (e.g., the urogenital system, breasts, and skin).

Changes can also occur in bone. Osteoporosis is defined as a decreased amount of bony tissue per unit volume of bone, leading to structural weakness. With lowered estrogen levels, there appears to be a decrease in osteoblast function and an increase in bone resorption. This leads to a structural weakness in bone and increases the risk of fracture. The most common sites of fracture are the radius, the neck of the femur, and the vertebral spine (Fig. 132).

Cardiovascular disease also increases with the lowered estrogen levels of the menopause. An increase in total cholesterol and low-density lipoprotein cholesterol occurs, along with a decline in high-density lipoprotein. Although these lipid changes account for increased risk, other factors such as changes in glucose tolerance and the direct effects of estrogen on arterial and venous blood flow are likely to be important.

Osteoporosis is described as the "silent epidemic" in that the disease may not be detected until the woman falls and fractures her osteoporotic bone(s). Wedge fractures of the spine may be detected on radiography (Fig. 133) and if multiple, may produce the "dowager's hump".

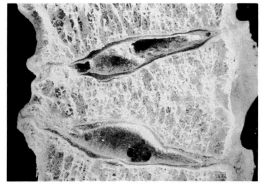

Fig. 132 Postmortem specimen of osteoporotic wedge fracture.

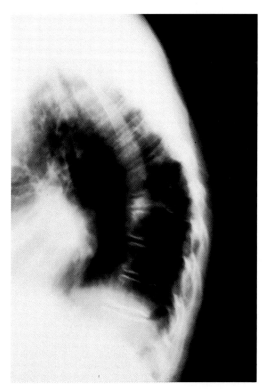

Fig. 133 Radiograph showing wedge fracture of thoracic spine.

17 / Menopause and climacteric

Clinical features	Hot flushes and night sweats are the classic symptoms of the menopause. Other symptoms include depression, vaginal soreness, vaginal dryness, urinary frequency, headaches, and joint pains. On examination, hair loss, dry skin, and vaginal atrophy may be present.
Investigations	If the diagnosis is in doubt, an FSH level of >15 IU/L will confirm ovarian failure.
	Noninvasive methods are now available to assess bone density. Single photon absorptiometry was initially used, then dual photon, and now dual-energy X-rays are used as the radioactive source (DXA, Fig. 134). Bone densitometry results of the hip are shown in Figure 135.
	Blood pressure, breasts, and cervical cytology should be checked as indicated. Mammography should be considered.
Management	Hormone replacement therapy (HRT) is the most appropriate treatment for women with menopause-related problems, osteoporosis prevention, and cardiovascular protection. Calcium supplementation is also advised.
	There are various methods of administration (Fig. 136).
	Oral. Estrogen tablets are given continuously and progestogen tablets are given for 12 days of each calendar month. For postmenopausal women (i.e., 1 year since last menstrual period), continuous combined preparations of estrogen and progestogen can be used to avoid monthly bleeding.
	Parenteral. Transdermal patches or estrogen creams are available. Estradiol implants can be inserted subcutaneously every 6 months; a testosterone implant may be inserted at the same time if the woman is sexually active, to improve libido. Creams, pessaries, or rings provide local treatment when used in the vagina.
	With all the above preparations, progestogens must be given if there is a uterus.
Complications	HRT has been connected with an increased risk of carcinoma. These claims are largely unfounded, although there may be a small increased risk of carcinoma of the breast with prolonged therapy (i.e., after 5–10 years).

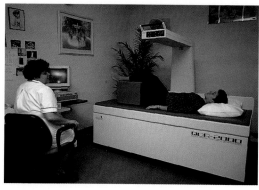

Fig. 134 Bone density measurement being performed.

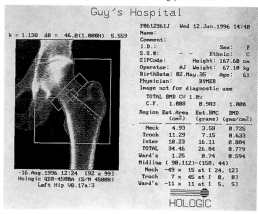

Fig. 135 DXA printout of bone density.

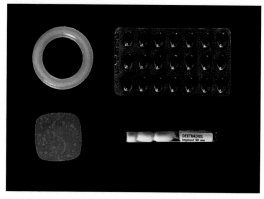

Fig. 136 HRT—implant, patch, oral tablets, vaginal ring.

Definition

The anterior vaginal wall is supported by the pubocervical fascia. This extends from the back of the symphysis pubis to the cervix and upper vagina. The posterior vaginal wall is supported by fibrous tissue of the rectovaginal septum and the levator ani muscles. The uterus is supported mainly by the cardinal or transverse cervical ligaments, which merge with the uterosacral ligaments before joining the cervix.

Uterovaginal prolapse is the downward displacement of the uterus (Fig. 137) and/or vagina toward or through the introitus. The bladder, urethra, rectum, and bowel may also be involved.

Vaginal wall prolapse

A prolapse of the lowest one-third of the anterior vagina involves the urethra and is called a urethrocoele. Prolapse of the upper two-thirds of the anterior vaginal wall involves the bladder and is therefore called a cystocele (Fig. 138). When the lower portion of the posterior vaginal wall prolapses, it brings with it the rectum and is therefore termed a rectocele. Prolapse of the vaginal wall above this involves the pouch of Douglas; it is called an enterocele (Fig. 139).

Etiology

Uncommon in nulliparous women, where it is due to congenital weakness of the pelvic supporting structures. The majority of women with prolapse have had children. Childbirth is associated with damage to the ligamentous tissues of the pelvis and nerve supply of the pelvic floor muscles, causing later weakness. Other factors contributing to or exacerbating these effects include postmenopausal atrophy of pelvic-supporting tissue and chronic raised intra-abdominal pressure (e.g., with obesity or chronic cough). ➡

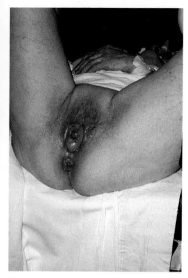

Fig. 137 Procidentia.

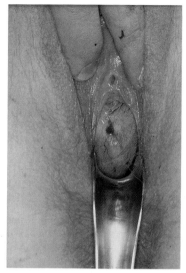

Fig. 138 Cystocele.

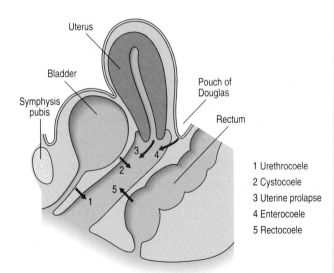

Fig. 139 Prolapse of the vagina.

1 Urethrocoele
2 Cystocoele
3 Uterine prolapse
4 Enterocoele
5 Rectocoele

Clinical features	Patients may describe a feeling of something "coming down," and there is the presence of a lump protruding through the vulva. Urinary incontinence may be associated with a urethrocele. Urinary retention may be seen when a large cystocele is present. Difficulty with defecation may also be present. Pain is not a feature of prolapse, but dragging discomfort and backache that worsen throughout the day may be experienced.
Management	*Prophylaxis:* Avoid traumatic vaginal deliveries and encourage antenatal and postnatal pelvic floor exercises. Discourage cigarette smoking and use HRT appropriately in postmenopausal women.
	Conservative treatment. Rings and shelf pessaries (Fig. 140) are a suitable short-term option in women unfit or not keen to undergo surgery and between pregnancies.
	Surgery. Procedures include the following: • *Anterior repair* corrects a cystocele but may not be the most appropriate treatment for stress incontinence. • *Posterior repair* corrects a rectocele. • *Vaginal hysterectomy* is the treatment of choice in uterine prolapse and is combined with anterior and posterior repairs as necessary (Fig. 141). • *Manchester (Fothergill) repair* involves shortening the transverse cervical ligaments and amputating the cervix, together with an anterior repair. It is a useful operation when the uterine body is well supported, but the cervix is elongated and protruding. A vaginal vault prolapse occurring after hysterectomy can be corrected by a sacrospinous fixation or by securing the vagina to the sacrum abdominally or laparoscopically.
Complications	Long-term use of pessaries can cause vaginal ulceration. Immediate complications of vaginal surgery include hemorrhage, hematoma formation, infection, and urinary retention. Wound breakdown and extrusion of bowel through the vagina (Fig. 142) are extremely rare. In the longer term, stenosis and dyspareunia may result. Prolapse may also recur.

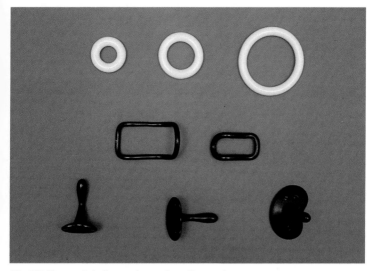

Fig. 140 Rings and shelf pessaries used to relieve prolapse.

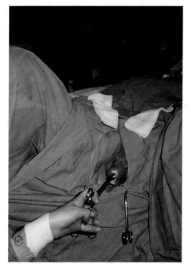

Fig. 141 Procidentia at commencement of vaginal hysterectomy.

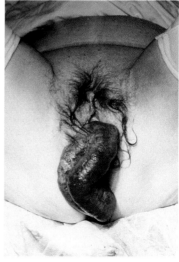

Fig. 142 Bowel herniation—a rare complication of vaginal hysterectomy.

Urge incontinence

Definition

Involuntary loss of urine caused by uninhibited detrusor contractions.

Etiology

Most cases are idiopathic. The detrusor contracts in an uninhibited fashion, causing urgency and frequency, and when the intravesical pressure exceeds the intraurethral pressure, incontinence results.

Clinical features

The history will reveal urinary frequency, urgency, nocturia, and perhaps, incontinence. On examination, there is usually no abnormality.

Investigations

A midstream urine specimen should be taken for microscopy and culture. If there is any suggestion of a "mixed picture" (i.e., symptoms of urge as well as stress), urodynamic investigations are essential (Fig. 143). Pad weighing can be used to assess incontinence. Videocystourethography is also useful (Fig. 144).

Management

Bladder drill. This requires patient motivation and ideally biofeedback. The patient is told to pass urine at certain time intervals, which are then gradually increased until 3 or 4 h is reached.

Drug therapy. Calcium antagonists, anticholinergic agents, ganglion blockers, estrogen replacement, and postganglion blockers.

Surgery. Clam cystoplasty, bladder transection, and sacral neurectomy are rarely used and are reserved for difficult cases.

Complications

Recurrence of symptoms is common. Bladder rupture can occur with cystodistension. Voiding difficulties can occur after surgery.

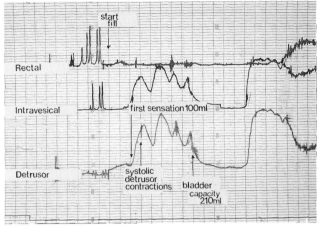

Fig. 143 Cystometry readout showing a stable bladder.

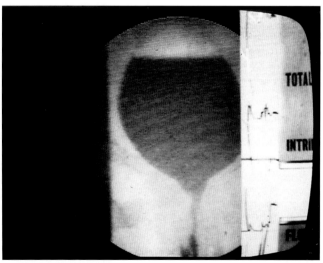

Fig. 144 Leakage of urine into bladder neck seen on videocystourethrography.

Genuine stress incontinence

Definition

Involuntary loss of urine when intra-abdominal pressure rises.

Etiology

Urethral sphincter weakness that is either congenital or secondary to multiparity, prolapse, menopause, or previous surgery.

Clinical features

The patient gives a history of losing urine involuntarily when she laughs, coughs, or sneezes. On examination, the vulva may be excoriated due to persistent wetness. If the patient is placed in the Sims position and a Sims speculum is inserted to display the anterior vaginal wall, urine loss may be demonstrated when the patient is asked to cough (providing her bladder is not empty). A cystocele may be present.

Management

Infection should be treated. Other treatments include:
- *Physiotherapy* involving pelvic floor exercises with cones (Fig. 145) or Faradism can be effective.
- *Colposuspension*. The bladder neck is elevated by inserting sutures beside the urethra and bladder neck. This can be done by using an abdominal incision or laparoscopically (Fig. 146).
- *Anterior colporrhaphy*. The urethra is elevated from below after opening up the anterior vaginal wall.
- *Slings*. Organic or inorganic material is used.
- *Endoscopic bladder neck suspensions*. This is useful for recurrent stress incontinence.
- *Artificial sphincters*.

Complications

Following surgery, voiding difficulties are common and recurrence of the stress incontinence is not uncommon. The results of surgery are poor if detrusor instability was present originally.

Prognosis

Colposuspensions have a 90% cure rate and anterior colporrhaphies 40–60%.

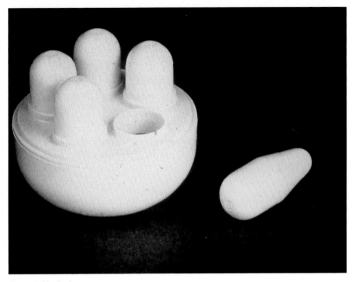

Fig. 145 Vaginal cones.

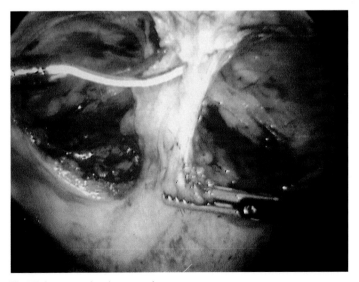

Fig. 146 Laparoscopic colposuspension.

Overflow incontinence

Frequent involuntary loss of small volumes of urine, slow urinary stream, and a postmicturition feeling of incomplete emptying.

Etiology   Obstruction to bladder outflow in bladder atony, which can be due to motor neuron lesions, drugs, surgery, pelvic mass, uterovaginal prolapse, local inflammation, or immobilization.

Clinical features   History will reveal the above symptoms. Examination will demonstrate an enlarged bladder, and catheterization will produce a large residual volume of urine.

Investigations   Midstream urine.

Cystometry. This will demonstrate a delayed first sensation and a large bladder capacity. Maximum voiding pressure will be normal or increased, and the peak flow rate will be slow. Micturating cystourethrogram (Fig. 147). Uroflowmeter.

Treatment   This will depend on the cause. Neurologic causes are not treatable, and intermittent self-catheterization can be learned.

True incontinence

Definition   Continuous incontinence.

Etiology   Usually due to a fistulous track (Fig. 148) secondary to obstructed labor, surgery, carcinoma, or radiotherapy.

Clinical features   There will be a history of continuous draining of urine from vagina. Examination may reveal the track, and coloring the urine may aid location.

Investigations   A micturating cystourethrogram and/or an IVP may help location.

Management   *Conservative:*   depending on etiology, some may heal with time.

Surgery: can be performed abdominally or vaginally. The fistulous track is removed, and an interposition graft may be used if the tissues are poor.

Complications   Stress incontinence, vaginal scarring, and recurrence.

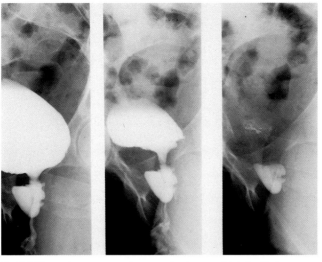

Fig. 147 Micturating cystogram demonstrating large urethral diverticulum.

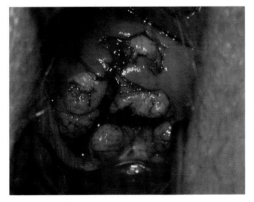

Fig. 148 Bladder mucosa visible through irregular fragments of vaginal mucosa.

Index